The CONNECT Framework®

CONNECT
First

Helping children and young people thrive through real-life communication

SUSANNAH BURDEN

BSc (Hons), PgDip AVT, LSLS Cert AVT

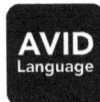

AVID
Language

Table of Contents

Foreword

When Susannah Burden, or Susie as I know her, first approached me with the idea for this book based on her CONNECT Framework, my first reaction was to feel flattered, and even a little confused, for here was this person whom I respected so much, even regarded with some awe to be honest, asking *me* for advice. From a personal perspective, it felt back-to-front... but the CONNECT approach, which nurtures the foundations underpinning communication, immediately struck a chord with me and, as the concept for a book, it felt just right.

Susie was the lead Auditory Verbal Therapist who taught me how to teach my profoundly deaf daughter to speak. How she and her fellow therapists changed my daughter's life – our whole family's life - is hard to put into words. It's also fair to say that we have worked with many other incredible professionals on this journey, not least the teachers at my daughter's school, her surgeons, audiologists and teachers of the deaf, but one thing is for sure: we would not be where we are today without the years we spent on that Auditory Verbal Therapy programme, under the guidance of Susie and her colleagues.

One of the things which initially attracted my husband and me to Auditory Verbal Therapy was its aspirational approach, which is also embodied in the CONNECT Framework. When your child first receives a diagnosis of "difference" (in our case profound deafness), the language around you changes – it becomes the language of limitation. With the best will in the world, people start to put your child in a box. "She is doing well *for a deaf child*" is a classic example. But we don't want our little girl to do well "for a deaf child" - we want her to be happy, to develop, to thrive *as an individual.*

Our very first exploratory conversation with an Auditory Verbal Therapist felt so different. Instead of telling us what our child wouldn't be able to do, the first question we were asked was, "What do you want for your daughter?". And then we were assured that, together with our therapists, we could work towards that goal. It wasn't a guarantee of what the future would hold or what the path would look like, but it was a guarantee that we would reach for the upper limits of our daughter's (still unknown) potential. And doesn't this make so much sense? Because, no matter who we are, whether or not we have "a diagnosis" of one kind or another, we are all individuals. We all have different horizons. And surely, for every one of us, it's worth reaching for that horizon, wherever it may lie. Who knows, we may even exceed it! Certainly, in our family's case, we are not going to put limits on our daughter's potential before she has even begun to really live her life. We are determined to give her the same opportunities as her hearing twin sister – in our family, at school, in friendships, in her professional career, in her relationships as an adult.

So, when Susie explained that she had been developing the CONNECT Framework, expanding out the principles that worked so well with deaf children, applying them to children, teens and young adults who were not deaf too – who communicated in all different ways, not just with speech - and combining these lessons with what she had seen working (while equally observing what was not working) over many years in her private practice as a Speech and Language Therapist, it resonated with me.

Even before seeing it formulated so brilliantly in this book, I have experienced the principles of this approach working within my own family. So much of what Susie taught me all those years ago, I have applied universally, both with my daughter who is deaf and my daughter who is not. Putting parents at the centre and in the driving seat of their child's individualised development, prioritizing connection over the headlong pursuit of communication (which naturally develops as a biproduct of connection and safety), and putting progress which can't be measured on a par with the milestones which can – this is a powerful combination.

Turning everyday routines into opportunities to connect deeply with your child is a key tenet of the CONNECT Framework. Reading Susie's suggestion of using a daily activity like breakfast as an opportunity for nurturing connection and communication reminded me of this photo (shown overleaf), one of my all-time favourites.

I was using the familiar, simple act of buttering toast as a shared point of connection with my daughter – she was spreading the butter (as best she could) while I was singing (as best I could), *"Spread, spread, spread the butter on the toast"*. At that point, my daughter only had a few spoken words, but look at her wholehearted engagement, with her smiling face upturned towards me. The trust. The safety. The joy.

This photo speaks a thousand words. This photo shows why connection is so important as the bedrock on which communication can grow.

Susie is courageous in her new endeavour to launch the CONNECT Framework out into the world, because it would have been easy to just keep doing what she has always done, and ignore the lessons she was learning along the way. After all, she was very successful at it. Being able to admit there are elements of what she has seen, learned and coached over many years which can be expanded and applied more widely, as well as elements of her practice which can be adapted to become even more effective bears testament to her commitment to the families she works with.

As a therapist, Susie has the courage of her convictions too. I remember the day she had to tell me that my daughter was not making the speech progress that would normally be expected by that point. This is not an easy discussion to have with a parent who has poured their all into supporting their child's progress – to have to say, "I'm not sure our current approach is working, despite everything you're doing, all the hard work, the days and hours spent driving back and forth to therapy, despite your child working her little socks off" - to have to suggest a change of direction, a starting all over again. But Susie also listened to me, as the parent, on that day. When I said we were seeing indicators of progress, but only at home (my daughter's safe place, with her safe people), Susie didn't dismiss my observations. When I said I believed the Auditory Verbal Therapy was working, but we just weren't seeing it play out in our scheduled therapy sessions yet, she listened. And when I said we wanted to continue for another six months before reviewing the situation again, she trusted my judgement. And I trusted her and the other therapists working with my daughter to come with us wholeheartedly and continue to guide us for those next six months. (And the rest, as they say, is history, for my daughter turned a corner shortly thereafter and her progress since then has taken our breath away.) This mutual trust between professionals and parents lies at the heart of the CONNECT Framework, and is one of the key principles that make it such a powerful approach.

One of the things which renders this book so useful is not only its detailed explanation of what underpins the CONNECT Framework – Susie's dual experience as a professional and as a parent walking a parallel path – but also the practical guidance she gives us. As parents, we are constantly bombarded with "Do this, do that, try this" to drive our child's progress forward. And, so often in response, we are left inwardly screaming, "But how? I understand the reasoning for doing it, but *HOW DO I ACTUALLY DO IT?*". Please don't miss the Appendices at the end of this book (and refer to them as you move through the chapters) because here Susie gives you sample scripts and real-world examples to help you put her guidance into practice in the real world. Using these as your starting point, you'll find it easier to build and adapt from there, to suit each individual situation as it arises in your own home and with your own family.

If you're in the thick of it right now, please know you're not alone. So many of us have been there too, and it's not easy – but it *is* worth it. Looking back on those early years, I can now see that what Susie says in this book was true for me at the time – and will be true for you too: **"You don't have to be perfect. You just have to show up... You're already doing more right than you think."**

~ *Tanya Saunders*
  Mother, wife, founder of AVID Language

Introduction

What if supporting your child's communication didn't mean squeezing in more therapy, more strategies, or more pressure—but instead meant noticing what's already there, and building on it?

This belief inspired me to create the CONNECT Framework—a relationship-first, neurodiversity-affirming approach that helps families support their child's communication, emotional regulation, and confidence in the moments that matter most.

Drawing from lived experience on both sides of the table—as a professional speech and language therapist, and as a mother—I invite you, fellow practitioners and parents, into a more compassionate, functional way of working with children and young people of all ages. Whether they are speaking or not yet using words, autistic, deaf, anxious, sensory-seeking, or simply wired differently, this book will help you understand what's going on beneath the surface and how to support growth through everyday routines and real-life connection.

You won't find pressure, perfection, or step-by-step scripts here. Instead, you'll find clarity, practical ideas, and a reminder that what your child needs most... is you.

Before you begin: What CONNECT stands for

This book is built around one core idea: **connection first.**

The CONNECT Framework gives families and professionals a way to support communication, regulation, and development in a way that feels natural, respectful, and sustainable.

Connection is always the starting point. It's what makes children feel safe enough to learn and engage. But connection isn't possible without a regulated nervous system. Regulation is the foundation that allows connection to grow. And from that connection, authentic communication can flourish.

In simple terms:

▶ **Regulation provides the base.**

▶ **Connection is the bridge.**

▶ **Communication is the outcome.**

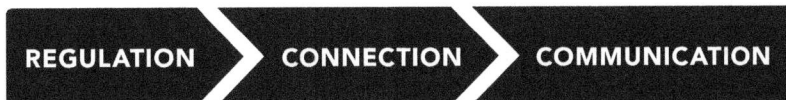

Each letter of CONNECT represents a principle that can guide our decisions, even in moments of uncertainty.

Let's start there:

C Connection First

Before anything else—goals, strategies, outcomes—we prioritise relationship and regulation. That's where communication begins.

O Observe and Adapt

We notice what's really happening, not just what's expected. We respond flexibly, based on what each child shows us.

N Natural Routines

Real-life moments are the best therapy. We work with the day-to-day, not around it.

N Neurodiversity-Affirming Practice

We honour each child's unique wiring and support their autonomy, not conformity.

E Empowered Caregivers

Families are not passive observers—they're the experts and co-leaders in their child's journey.

C Communication as an Outcome of Regulation

We don't force language. We support emotional safety, so communication can emerge naturally.

T Togetherness

Not just with the child—but with the whole team around the child. True progress happens when everyone is on the same page, working *with* each other rather than in isolation.

You don't need to memorise all of this now. You'll see it unfold, one chapter at a time. But keep this in mind: **when we focus on connection, communication follows.**

Read this first: The power of showing up

If you're reading this, chances are you care deeply about your child or the children/ young people you support. You want to do the right thing. You want to get it *right*. But here's something we don't say often enough:

You don't have to be perfect. You just have to show up.

Family life is messy. Regulating a toddler mid-tantrum or trying to connect with a teenager who's barely speaking—none of it looks like a textbook. Most of the time, you're doing the best you can with the energy and capacity you've got in that moment. That **counts**. In fact, that's exactly what this book is about.

This isn't a model built on perfection. It's built on **progress**.

Even a 5% shift—one pause before reacting, one tiny moment of connection—can make a meaningful difference to your child's development. Every one of those moments is like a penny in the bank. Small deposits, over time, become something powerful.
And if you've ever talked yourself out of trying because you thought "I won't be able to do this every time"—know this:

That's your brain trying to protect you from feeling that you're failing.

But you're not failing.

You're here. You're reading. You're investing in your relationship with your child in a more meaningful way than you probably realise.

Let go of perfect. Let go of pressure.

Connection grows in the ordinary, imperfect moments.

An Open Letter to Professionals

Dear Fellow Professionals,

If you're reading this book as a therapist, teacher, assistant, caseworker, or any kind of professional supporting children, young people and families—welcome. I'm so glad you're here.

Although this book is written primarily with parents in mind, I want to be clear from the outset: **your expertise, your training, and your insight are deeply valued**. I've sat in your chair. I know the weight you carry, the care you give, and the frustration that can come when the system feels like it gets in the way of the work you trained to do.

The CONNECT Framework isn't about replacing what you already know. It's about offering a shift in lens—not a rejection of practice, but an expansion of it.

At its heart, CONNECT is a **complementary approach**. It sits alongside the structured methods, evidence-based interventions, and tools you already use—not in competition with them. If anything, it helps those tools land more effectively in a child's natural world by strengthening the bridge between professional insight and everyday life.

This book may read as if it speaks directly to parents—but you're invited into that space, too. My hope is that it encourages you to look at your own work with fresh eyes:

▶ How do we empower caregivers rather than instruct them?

▶ How can our diagnostic skill and clinical reasoning filter into the tiny, unmeasured moments that shape a child's development?

▶ What happens when we value presence just as much as progress?

I know many professionals are working within rigid systems—IEP, ISP or EHCP deadlines, staffing gaps, tick-box targets, and limited time. This book doesn't ignore those realities. Instead, it gently asks whether the **moments that can't be measured** might still hold the most meaning.

Throughout the chapters, I've included reflection questions that are designed not just for parents, but also for you. You might find them worded for caregivers—but many are easily reframed.

Where a parent is invited to ask, "When do I feel most connected to my child?", you might ask: "When do I feel most aligned with this family?".

Or instead of "Where can I ease pressure?" perhaps: "Where might I unintentionally be creating pressure?"

I hope this book gives you not only a practical framework to share with families, but also an affirmation of what you're already doing—and the encouragement to be human, curious, and adaptive in your practice.

We know that when we work in partnership with parents to provide something flexible, diagnostic and individualised, then therapy can carry over into day-to-day life and **children thrive.**

Thank you for reading,

Susannah

Chapter One

The Starting Line

What singing, therapy, and parenthood taught me about connection

I've always found children fascinating. There's something about the moment they let you into their world—when you follow their lead and, suddenly, you're included in something that matters and is important to them. Even as a teenager, I loved being part of that spark, that creativity. Whether it was babysitting for families I knew, helping out in schools, or volunteering at Sunday school at our local Methodist Church, it always felt natural to tune in and connect. Even back then, I think I was drawn to the way children communicate beyond just words.

I come from a long line of teachers, and although that world felt familiar, when the time came to choose a career, I found myself drawn elsewhere. I'd spent years training in voice and performance as a semi-professional folk singer. Singing lessons taught me about the incredible power of the voice—how you can shape sound, direct emotion, and connect with others just by controlling breath and pitch. It was fascinating. The voice wasn't just a tool; it was a bridge. And alongside that, I had always loved language, even though—like many dyslexic people—I'd once felt I didn't "belong" in the world of words.

Speech and language therapy felt like the perfect intersection of those things: creativity, communication, and connection. Still, the idea of a degree full of reading and theory was daunting. But with the right support, I found ways to learn that made sense to me. I took English Language as an A-level, leaned into what worked for me, and gave myself permission not to fear the parts that didn't.

During my undergraduate training, I worked across a range of settings—voice clinics, early intervention, and cancer services—but I always felt most at home with the little ones. Something about early years—the wildness and rawness and honesty—just made sense to me.

Then I saw the job advert.

A trainee position as an *Auditory Verbal Therapist*. I didn't know then how much that opportunity would shape not only my work, but my entire way of seeing children, families, and communication itself.

Learning to listen differently

The training to become an Auditory Verbal Therapist was intense—possibly one of the steepest learning curves of my life. I had to learn how to coach in the moment, to be present, diagnostic, to observe and problem-solve on the fly. There were wobbles, for sure—moments I thought I'd never get it, times I felt completely out of my depth. But I was lucky. I had mentors who truly believed in what this approach could do.

Jacqueline Stokes trained under Daniel Ling and brought this approach to the UK at a time when it was virtually unknown. Her passion, energy, and absolute belief in parents' power to change their child's communication trajectory was infectious—and, at times, a little intimidating. I also learned from therapists like Catherine White, Elizabeth Tyszkiewicz, Rosie Quayle, and Donna Sperandio. Each of them shaped me in different ways. Each of them taught me something about how to listen, how to coach, and how to stay with families in the hard moments.

One thing that stood out to me early on was how families would travel *across the country* for their one-hour, **fortnightly** session. This was completely foreign to me. I'd always been taught that therapy should be frequent—ideally weekly, if not more. Surely one hour every two weeks wasn't enough?

But I quickly came to understand something that changed everything: the most important learner in the room wasn't the child—it was the parent.

That hour wasn't the "therapy". The therapy happened **in between** the sessions—when the parent took what they had learned and wove it into the fabric of everyday life. This principle changed the way I saw progress. And it's something I still repeat to the families I work with now.

It wasn't a drop-off clinic. Parents didn't come in, leave their child with a therapist, and pop off to the shops or for a coffee. No—parents were absolutely essential to every single session. They were present, engaged, and learning in real time. I remember one family who drove from the Scottish Highlands to Glasgow, caught a flight to Birmingham, then hired a car to get to Oxford for their session. Every two weeks. That was their routine. Because they believed—rightly—that it was working. That it was *changing* things.

Families came from Europe. From all corners of the UK. And still, that hour wasn't too short, and the fortnight wasn't too long. Because they left with something more powerful than a worksheet—they left with clarity, confidence, and the *why* behind every interaction they were being coached to try.

One of the most powerful examples for me was a trilingual family I supported. They were raising twin boys who were profoundly deaf in the UK. Understandably, the parents asked: *Which language should we focus on? Should we drop some? Just do English?* And the beauty of the parent coaching model was that it didn't require us to dictate a "right answer". Instead, we gave them tools they could apply across all three languages.

By the time those boys started school, they were speaking all three languages fluently. In fact, according to the assessments we used, they were **ahead** in English—and one of the boys made twenty-four months of language progress in just six months. But again, this wasn't about the therapist "doing a brilliant job". It was about how powerfully the parents embraced the learning; how much they applied it across real-life situations. That's where the magic was.

Dyslexia, fear, and finding my own voice

And perhaps one reason I've always connected with parents trying to navigate a system that doesn't always fit, is because I know that feeling myself.

As a child, I took longer than others to learn to read. I assumed it was because I just wasn't very bright. I vividly remember being in GCSE English, dreading the part of the lesson when the teacher would ask us to read aloud. I'd count ahead—desperately trying to work out which pages might land in my lap— just so I could prepare and not stumble in front of everyone.

That fear froze me. Literally. My brain would go offline. I was in a freeze response—totally dysregulated, flooded with self-doubt. In those moments, I couldn't learn. I couldn't think clearly. And it didn't matter how intelligent I was, or wasn't—I couldn't access the learning because I was not regulated.

Eventually, I found the courage to speak to my English teacher. I explained that reading aloud was something I really struggled with. To his credit, he agreed to let me opt out. And suddenly, something shifted. I could focus. I could actually listen, absorb the story, engage with the lesson. And I ended up (somewhat surprisingly) getting an A* in English Literature—not because I'd suddenly become more intelligent, but because I'd finally been given the environment I needed in order to learn.

That experience taught me something I carry with me every day: we don't need "special needs" labels to justify making learning accessible. We need **individual understanding**. Everyone has a different doorway to learning. We just need the space, support, and autonomy to walk through it.

On both sides of the table

A few years after becoming a parent for the second time, I began to notice that one of my children processed the world a little differently. Everyday experiences sometimes felt overwhelming for them in ways I couldn't immediately understand.

As a therapist, I instinctively began tracking developmental milestones, analysing play, and reaching for checklists. But in doing so, I missed the most important part: the little person in front of me.

What they needed wasn't more analysis—they needed me. They needed co-play, safety, and space. And when I finally stepped into their world without an agenda, something shifted. Their communication began to blossom—not because I worked harder, but because I connected with them.

I had been so focused on ticking boxes that I had forgotten to really engage with their thinking and emotions. I wanted to get them speaking more—but they needed me to *understand* more. They needed to play. To be seen. To feel safe. I realised I'd fallen into the very trap I often supported parents out of: trying to "fix" communication instead of fostering *relationship*.

When I paused, joined their world, and let go of my agenda—that's when things changed. We began to play, to imagine, to co-create. And their language? It bloomed. Not because I pushed harder, but because I finally stopped pushing at all.

The moment everything came together

It was this personal journey—learning to apply the principles of Auditory Verbal Therapy within a neurodiversity-affirming, connection-first framework—that cracked something open in me.

Suddenly, I could see how this could work far beyond deafness. Yes, AVT was rooted in developing listening pathways in the brain, but its core strength was something deeper: coaching, co-regulation, responsive interaction, and trust in the parent-child relationship.

And so, I stepped into independent practice.

It was terrifying. Would people understand what I was offering? Was my approach too niche? I was even advised by one therapist to "stay in my lane".

But what they didn't necessarily understand was that my lane wasn't narrow at all—it was broad and winding and built on decades of experience, not just with families of deaf children, but with anyone who needed a different way in. Because what makes AVT powerful isn't just the listening—it's the way it holds parents at the centre. Principle 4 of the Auditory Verbal approach—

"Guide and coach parents to become the primary facilitators of their child's listening and spoken language development through active, consistent participation in individualised auditory verbal therapy"—is more than a professional standard. It's the heartbeat of this work. It helps you spot the invisible blockers, reframe what you see, and unlock real, functional connection through everyday moments.

That's how the CONNECT Framework was born.

Reflection

For the Reader

If you're reading this as a parent, especially one who feels unsure or overwhelmed, I want you to know:
This is not just my story. It's yours, too. Your experiences, instincts, and insights matter.

Here are some gentle questions to reflect on:

1. Have you ever felt pressure to tick developmental boxes, rather than tune into what your child really needs?

2. In what moments do you feel most connected to your child?

3. Are there parts of your parenting journey that surprised you—things you thought you'd "know" but had to learn differently?

4. What are your biggest strengths as a parent (even if they feel hidden)?

5. What would it mean to trust your own instincts more?

For Professionals: reflecting on practice

▶ What moments in my professional life have reminded me why I chose this work?

▶ When have I felt most aligned with a parent, even before progress was visible?

Chapter Two

Where The Lane Splits

When a specialist approach becomes a universal need

When I first started working as an Auditory Verbal Therapist, I believed—like most people—that this was a specialist approach, designed for a very specific group: deaf children with access to auditory input. It made sense. After all, the entire model centred on activating and strengthening the listening brain.

But the longer I worked in that space, the more I began to question the boundaries we had drawn around it. Not because the approach wasn't specific or precise—it absolutely was—but because at its *core*, it was something much more universal. It was about the power of responsive interaction. It was about coaching parents to notice, adapt, and connect in real time. It was about helping a child's *whole brain*—not just the auditory pathways—make sense of the world.

The families I saw weren't just teaching their children to hear—they were building trust, co-regulation, shared joy, and confidence through everyday experiences. The same things that so many other families needed, too.

What if this wasn't only for deaf children?

It started as a quiet question in the back of my mind: *What if these principles could help children beyond those who are deaf?* What if the true magic wasn't just in the hearing aids or cochlear implants—but in the *parent-child relationship itself?*

I was working with families who were incredibly tuned-in, reflective, and engaged. They weren't coming to therapy to be taught how to *do* things for their children. They were learning how to *be* with them—differently, more intentionally, with greater clarity and less pressure.

They were learning to:

- ► Pause and observe, instead of jumping in
- ► Follow their child's lead, even when it wasn't where they expected
- ► Use natural routines as opportunities for learning
- ► Speak with purpose, not just frequency
- ► Let go of the urge to fix, and tune into their child's thought process instead.

And I started wondering—*why don't we teach this to all families?* Not just those with deafness, or speech delays, or a diagnosis. Just families. Parents. Humans.

Leaving the lane (or so they thought)

When I began taking these ideas beyond their original setting, I encountered some resistance—not from families, but from the wider system. From other professionals.

There was a sense that what I was doing belonged in a very specific box. That it was too specialist, or perhaps too different to apply more broadly, and couldn't possibly be of benefit to clients who weren't deaf.

But my work had never been about ticking boxes. It had always been about coaching, listening deeply, spotting the invisible blockers that hold children—and parents—

back. It was about responding in the moment and supporting families to take small, meaningful steps forward.

What others hadn't yet seen was that this wasn't a fringe idea. It was a universal truth, hiding in plain sight within specialist practice. To limit this work to one setting or one group would be to close the door on exactly the families who needed it most.

When the system doesn't fit

I felt inspired to begin working independently, supporting a range of families—toddlers, teens, children with complex needs, those without a diagnosis but with very real challenges. And what I saw confirmed what I already knew: connection-first, coaching-based support worked.

It worked for parents who had felt dismissed or blamed.

It worked for children who didn't thrive in traditional therapy rooms.
It worked for families who were told to "wait and see," or who were passed from service to service without ever really being heard.

I supported one family with a teenage son who had stopped attending school due to anxiety. His parents were desperate for help but exhausted by conflicting advice and long waiting lists. We didn't start with a programme or checklist. We started by noticing—how he communicated when he felt safe, when he felt pressure, when he felt misunderstood.

Then we made small shifts. Conversations in the car. Changes to language that reduced demand. Moments of play that didn't have an outcome attached.

And that's when it clicked: **this isn't about therapy goals—it's about everyday connection.**

The family began to understand how their son processed information. They learned to step back when needed, and to lean in with curiosity, not correction. Slowly, his confidence returned. He began to engage again—not because we pushed harder, but because we created a space where he didn't need to guard himself.

I remember another child—a seven-year-old boy who arrived with just a handful of single words and frequent, violent dysregulation. His mum was heartbroken and overwhelmed. He would hit, kick, and spit when he was distressed, and she often felt helpless— especially as he got bigger and harder to physically contain.

Everyday life was unpredictable. The smallest things could trigger an explosion. Her greatest fear was not knowing how to help him feel safe.

But again, we didn't start with behaviour charts. We didn't try to manage or suppress the outbursts. We focused on understanding what he was trying to communicate beneath the behaviour. We built connection. We created safety.

And slowly, everything started to shift. His communication grew—from single words to phrases, and then to full sentences. The outbursts lessened, then faded altogether. His mum recently said she can't even remember the last time he lost control.

Now, he wraps his arms around her and says, *"Love you, Mum."*

That's what happens when we meet behaviour with curiosity instead of control. That's what happens when we *see* the child behind the dysregulation—and give them the space to show us who they really are.

Parents are not passive participants

One of the most powerful lessons I've carried with me from Auditory Verbal Therapy is this: **the most important work happens outside the room.**

It's not about the one-hour fortnightly sessions—it's about the 335 hours in between.

It's not about the worksheets or flashcards—it's about the breakfast table, the supermarket trip, the school run.
It's not about performance—it's about *presence.*

When parents are seen as co-creators of progress—not assistants to the professional—they unlock something powerful. And when they're coached with respect, clarity, and belief, they rise.

That's what I saw in AVT. That's what I see now in families across every kind of need. And that's what the CONNECT Framework is built on.

From compliance to connection

Traditional therapy often puts the child under the microscope: What are they doing? What aren't they doing? How do we get them to do more?

But the CONNECT Framework flips that lens. Instead of "What's missing?", we ask:

- What's meaningful to this child?
- What are they telling us, even without words?
- What's getting in the way of their communication—and how can we clear a path, together?

It's not about compliance. It's about **understanding**. It's not about fixing. It's about **connecting**. It's not about what a child can *do*—it's about *who they are*, and how we support their voice to grow, however that voice sounds.

Reflection

For the Reader

You too may have been advised to "stay in your lane" as a parent.

You may have been made to feel like your instincts don't count.

That your role is to follow instructions, not lead the way.

But here's what I want you to know:

- ► You know your child better than anyone.
- ► You're allowed to challenge what doesn't feel right.
- ► You're allowed to seek connection over correction.
- ► And you are *not* a passive participant in your child's growth.

So as you read this chapter, take a moment to reflect:

1. Have you ever felt boxed in by "the system" or told that your instincts weren't enough?

2. Are there times you've seen your child thrive when the pressure is removed?

3. What would it look like to make everyday connection your focus—not outcomes, not expectations?

4. What's your "lane"? And does it still fit, or are you ready to step into something new?

For Professionals: reflecting on practice

▶ Are there areas where rigid systems have shaped my practice more than I'd like?

▶ How might I bring more flexibility into my work without losing structure?

APPENDIX SUGGESTION

<u>Appendix A:</u>
The CONNECT Framework Summary
It might be helpful to look at the summary now in order to consider the universal relevance of this approach.

Chapter Three

Not Just Toddlers

Why the CONNECT approach works with teens too

When we talk about communication support, early years often get the spotlight. And rightly so—those first few years of life are incredibly important. Between birth and seven, the brain is at its most malleable. In fact, from birth to age three, neuroplasticity is at its most sensitive. The brain is primed to shape and wire itself based on the input it receives, and early intervention—especially when it comes to language and auditory pathways—can make a huge difference.

But somewhere along the line, that truth has been misinterpreted.

We've developed this quiet, collective belief that if a child hasn't made progress by the time they reach school age, or if connection feels fractured by the teenage years, then it's somehow "too late."

Let me be really clear: **it's not.**

The adolescent brain is still evolving

Teenagers are still developing—rapidly. They're moving into a time of huge neurological and emotional change. Their sense of identity is forming. Their brains are still pruning, still rewiring, still open to connection. And yes, the stakes feel different. They crave autonomy. They pull away from parents and towards peers. But even as they seek more independence, they still need us—desperately.

The parent-child relationship is evolving in these years. It can feel unfamiliar, even strained. But that evolution is rich with opportunity. We don't lose our influence as parents—we simply have to connect in new ways.

STORY: One Girl's Island

I once worked with a bright, insightful young lady who had relatively recently received a diagnosis of autism. She was articulate, reflective, and deeply self-aware—but struggling. School was a source of huge anxiety, and navigating friendships felt overwhelming and unpredictable.

At first, the goal was framed around "social communication"—understanding perspective, reading cues, supporting theory of mind.

But as we began to work together, the focus shifted. It became less about theory, and more about *regulation*. About *connection*.

She started to notice how her body felt when she was anxious. She could describe the way her thoughts spiralled, how her words sometimes stuck or vanished when things felt too much. Together, we explored her internal 'battery'—what charges it, what drains it, how her brain needed dopamine—how many neurodivergent people don't produce enough of it naturally, and how that lack affects everything from motivation to mood.

It's something I often share with parents: *connection relies on regulation, and regulation relies on safety*. We can't build communication skills on a foundation of stress. We have to work with the nervous system, not against it.

This young woman had a brilliant metaphor. She described her world as an island. Her

parents and siblings lived *on* the island—
her safe people. The rest of her life existed
around it:

- Fish were the people who flitted in and
  out—friendly, but passing.
- Lifeboats were those who circled nearby,
  offering support when needed.
- Sharks were those she didn't trust—people
  who triggered fear or guardedness.
- Jellyfish were the trickiest. They *looked*
  safe but could sting when she wasn't
  expecting it.

This island analogy became a springboard
for everything: how to build and protect
boundaries, how to tell the difference
between real connection and performance,
how to consider **her own role** in someone
else's island. *Am I a fish on their island? A
shark? A lifeboat?*

That kind of reflective, relational language
didn't come from a worksheet. It came from

a space of trust, and from honouring who she already was—not trying to change her, but helping her understand herself more deeply.

It's not about resources, it's about relevance

A lot of therapists (and parents) feel nervous about working with teenagers. It can feel like a completely different language. The games that worked in early years don't quite land. Printed social stories or structured group programmes can fall flat.

So, what do we do instead?

We start with *what matters to them*. One teenage boy I worked with loved YouTube. He was animated and expressive when he talked about his favourite creators. So that's where we began—by connecting through shared interest. We didn't ask him to stop doing what he loved to attend to "therapy."

We joined him in his world and looked for moments of connection *within* it.

With teens, therapy isn't about hoop-jumping. It's not about finishing a task or completing a target. It's about thinking diagnostically:

- ► Where is this young person now?
- ► Where do they want to be?
- ► What's in the way?
- ► What's my role in helping the parent and child unblock that path together?

Sometimes, that's about emotional literacy. Sometimes it's about executive functioning— helping them plan revision, organise their day, structure their language in an essay. Sometimes, it's about working with the parent to create a home environment that feels safe enough to *try* again.

It's never about fitting a child to a system. It's about adapting the system to the child.

From resistance to relationship

Adolescence is often framed as a time of resistance. And yes, it can feel that way—especially for parents. But resistance often masks vulnerability. What looks like defiance is often self-protection. What looks like apathy is sometimes exhaustion or overwhelm. What looks like manipulation may actually be fear.

Teenagers don't want to be managed. They want to be *met*.

That doesn't mean giving in. It means letting go of control as the main goal and choosing *relationship* instead.

Because here's what I've seen—again and again: when connection is secure, communication can grow. Even in teenagers. Even in young people who've shut down, tuned out, or lashed out.

And still... change happens

When we work through the CONNECT lens with teenagers, we often see changes that feel deeply emotional—because they are.

I've worked with young people who once screamed and kicked at the school gates, but now walk in on their own.

I've seen teenagers who once refused to speak, finding the words to explain their feelings—on their own terms.

I've seen teens who once pushed their parents away, now leaning in for a hug and wanting a chat.

And I've seen young people step into the

adult world with confidence—*not because they were suddenly ready*, but because someone helped them prepare in the right way.

One young man I supported in a college setting was on a pathway-to-employment programme. He had an upcoming internship with a national energy supplier, and while there was a real sense of excitement, there was also understandable anxiety. This wasn't just another placement—it came with the potential for real, long-term employment. He was determined to make the most of it.

But we had to be pragmatic. Real-world settings are full of unseen challenges—especially for neurodivergent young people. Navigating public transport. Switching between unfamiliar departments. Managing your own time. Fulfilling tasks in a professional environment. All of it takes communication, flexibility, emotional regulation, and executive functioning—and none of that should be left to chance.

So I worked closely with his placement coach to understand the nature of the role in detail. Together, we thought ahead. We anticipated what might come up and prepared for it. Because it's always easier to catch the ball when you can see it coming than to run after it once it's passed you by.

We practised social scripts for introductions and small talk. We explored how to write professional emails and how to structure requests. We talked about boundaries—what was expected of him, and what he could expect in return. We broke down his tasks into manageable, concrete chunks, and we rehearsed what to say and do in key moments.

Most importantly, *we didn't assume anything was obvious.* We treated every element of the placement as something worth teaching,

coaching, and preparing for—*on purpose.*
And we found ways for him to connect with
the people around him so that he could feel
not just competent, but safe.

And he thrived. He moved between
departments, contributed meaningfully,
and built relationships with people in the
workplace.
His confidence soared—not because we fixed
him, but because we *prepared* him.

That's the heart of CONNECT. It's not about
waiting for challenges to arise and then trying
to manage the fallout. It's about noticing
the likely blockers, equipping families to
support those areas in real life, and helping
young people experience success in the
environments they want to grow in.

This young man left his placement with
a clearer sense of his future—and more
importantly, belief in his own ability to be
part of it.

Reflection

For the Reader

Parenting a teenager is hard. You're watching your child pull away just when things feel most uncertain. But you haven't lost them. You're just learning a new way to walk alongside them.

Try sitting with these reflections:

1. What feels hard about connecting with your teen right now?

2. What helps you feel close—even briefly?

3. Are there signals or behaviours that might mean something deeper than what they appear?

4. What's one small shift you could make to offer more choice or shared problem-solving?

5. If your child could redesign the way you interact, what might they keep—and what might they gently ask to change?

For Professionals: reflecting on practice

▶ Do I feel equipped to support older children and teens through a relational lens?

▶ Where could I shift my approach to better meet a young person in their world?

APPENDIX SUGGESTION

Appendix J:

Supporting Your Young Person into Employment and Purpose

If you're thinking about next steps for your young person, this resource is for you.

Chapter Four

The Birth Of The CONNECT Framework

From professional tools to everyday transformation

It didn't come to me all at once. There was no lightbulb moment, no flash of brilliance over coffee or a post-it note on the fridge that suddenly made it clear. The CONNECT Framework emerged gradually, layer by layer, through years of listening, trying, wondering, and watching families grow—not just in therapy rooms, but in *real life*.

It grew in the middle of supermarket aisles

and bedtime meltdowns. It took shape in the moments when I paused in a session and realised, **this is what's actually working.** It came from the joy of a toddler finding their first phrase and the fierce pride of a teenager telling their parent, *"You finally get me."*

Most of all, it came from sitting on both sides of the table—as a therapist and as a parent.

The frustration that sparked a new way

For years, I felt the tension that so many therapists feel. I'd spend an hour with a family and pour everything I could into that time—strategies, modelling, guidance—and then they'd leave. And I'd wonder:

What will actually stick? What will feel useful tomorrow morning when the cereal spills and a school shoe is missing?

Too often, families left sessions feeling more pressure than clarity. The strategies were sound, but they didn't always translate. The language felt too clinical. The progress felt distant.

What families needed wasn't more jargon. It wasn't more exercises to "complete".

They needed a way to feel *anchored*. They needed to feel that how they lived, how they spoke, how they noticed and responded— *that* was enough to build something powerful.

And I realised: they didn't need a plan. They needed a framework.

CONNECT: A framework for everyday life

I didn't consciously set out to invent CONNECT. It evolved organically.

Over time, I began to recognise consistent threads—things I saw in families who made meaningful, lasting progress. And I wrote those things down. Over and over. They weren't always in order, and they weren't always neat. But together, they formed something that helped people remember what mattered most—even when things felt messy.

That became the CONNECT Framework.

CONNECT stands for:

C – Connection First

O – Observe and Adapt

N – Natural Routines

N – Neurodiversity-Affirming Practice

E – Empowered Caregivers

C – Communication as an Outcome of Regulation

T – Togetherness

Each of these phrases is more than a principle—they're threads you can return to again and again. When you're not sure what to do, when nothing's working, when you feel disconnected or disempowered—CONNECT gives you a way to come back to what really matters.

Let me tell you where each piece came from.

▶ *Connection First*

This one was never in doubt. I saw it from my earliest days as a therapist—nothing meaningful happens without connection. Not language. Not learning. Not growth. It's the safety net that holds it all.

But it became even more real when I was parenting my own children and realised that sometimes the *right* strategy didn't work—because the connection wasn't there. Or because they were dysregulated. Or because I was.

Connection isn't about being calm all the time. It's about *being present*. It's the heartbeat of every strong therapeutic relationship, and every safe family bond.

▶ *Observe and Adapt*

This came from the "aha" moments— those times I watched a parent's eyes light up because they suddenly *noticed* something new. A cue. A pattern. A point of dysregulation. A moment of enjoyment.

Observation sounds passive, but it's incredibly active. And when you pair it with adaptation—*what can I shift here?* —you become empowered. You stop trying to fit your child into a plan and start shaping the plan around your child.

This thread helped parents stop reacting and start *responding*. It became a core muscle of the framework.

▶ *Natural Routines*

The more families I supported, the more I realised: it's not about the scheduled therapy sessions. It's about all the hours in between.

Therapy can't only happen in therapy. It has to live in the walk to nursery, the bedtime routine, the moments spent sorting laundry or brushing teeth. These aren't time-fillers—they're language-rich, emotionally meaningful, high-context opportunities to connect and grow.

"Natural routines" gave families permission to let go of the Pinterest-worthy activities and lean into what they were already doing.

▶ *Neurodiversity-Affirming Practice*

One key thing I have learned over the years is that when you parent or work with a neurodivergent child, your lens shifts.

Suddenly, the strategies that once "worked" feel off-key. The goals you used to write feel misaligned. And your own instincts, long buried under training and standardisation, begin to rise again.

At times in my own parenting journey, I remember feeling lost—when things felt different, and I couldn't find the right lens to make sense of it… being a therapist, and feeling overwhelmed—unsure whether I was helping or hindering by adding too much pressure.

During a season when parenting felt especially uncertain, I was lucky to be visited by an inspirational and very knowledgeable colleague and friend. They quietly observed the rhythms of our afternoon, joined in play, and gently but firmly offered a sentence that stayed with me:

"Do not view your child through a deficit lens."

It landed like lightning.

That one line changed everything. It grounded me. It reminded me that different isn't broken. And it challenged me to parent from a place of connection and curiosity—not correction.

I carry that reminder with me in my work now, sharing it with other families and professionals. It's not a dismissal of challenge—it's an invitation to see children as they are, not as problems to solve.

That phrase became a mantra I still repeat to the parents I work with today. And not just with parents. It's a reminder to everyone in the room that we are not here to fix these young people. We are not here to treat their profile as a problem.

That is why I don't refer to autism as "autistic spectrum disorder". It's not a disorder that needs correcting or treating. It's a way of being that deserves understanding, support, and honour.

To affirm neurodiversity is to believe that there is no one "normal" brain to measure others against. It's to say: *You are not broken. You're wired differently—and your wiring is valid.*

This shift isn't just philosophical. It's practical. When we stop seeing a child's profile as something to fix, we stop trying to mould them to the environment—and instead, we start shaping the environment to meet them where they are and give them the tools and strategies to be the happiest most successful version of themselves. That's when real growth begins.

▶ *Empowered Caregivers*

Over the years, I've met so many parents—especially mothers—who arrived in sessions carrying a quiet weight. A sense that they were getting it wrong. That someone else—usually a professional—held the key to unlocking their child's potential.

But here's the truth: they were never the problem. And they never needed fixing either.

What they needed was recognition. Recognition of the deep, instinctive understanding they already had of their child. And space to be heard, trusted, and supported in that role.

Because when we stop seeing professionals as the sole experts and start seeing intervention as a meeting of minds—a partnership of expertise—everything shifts. Parents bring the day-to-day knowledge, the emotional insight, the context. Professionals bring tools, coaching, and perspective. And together, that's where the real progress happens.

When caregivers feel empowered, they stop performing for professionals and start truly partnering with their child. And that shift? It changes everything.

▶ *Communication as an Outcome of Regulation (and Connection)*

This came from watching years of therapy that tried to force communication before safety. And it just didn't work.

I saw children shut down, zone out, melt down—not because they couldn't learn, but because they didn't feel regulated. Their nervous systems were in survival mode.

The breakthrough came when I stopped chasing expressive language and started looking for the **conditions** that allowed communication to emerge. And every time, it circled back to regulation.

This thread became the foundation for my belief that communication is not just a goal. It's a *result*—and the pre-work matters more than we think.

▶ *Togetherness*

This final thread is simple but essential.
It's about shared experience. Shared wins.
Shared hard moments.

So many families arrive in therapy feeling isolated—like the work is on their shoulders alone. This piece of CONNECT reminds us that progress doesn't happen in silos. We need each other. Children need parents. Parents need therapists who listen. And communities that lift, not judge.

Togetherness is about walking this path *with*, not *for*. It's the glue that holds the framework together.

Why CONNECT works

I've used CONNECT with toddlers, teens, and children with profound and complex needs. I've used it with families navigating diagnosis, those in complete burnout, and those who just want to understand their child a little better.

It works not because it's prescriptive, but because it's *anchoring.* It gives you something to hold onto when everything else feels uncertain. It reminds you that language doesn't grow in pressure, and parenting doesn't have to look like perfection.

It reminds you that *you are already doing more right than you think.*

A framework, not a formula

If you take one thing from this chapter, let it be this: CONNECT is a way of seeing, not a checklist.

You don't need to apply it all at once. You don't need to master it before it "counts". You're probably already doing parts of it without even realising. This isn't something extra to do—it's a lens you can carry into what you're already doing.

In the next set of chapters, we'll walk through each thread of the CONNECT Framework in detail. You'll hear stories, try out practical ideas, and reflect on how it fits your child, your family, and your life.

But before we go there, take a moment to reflect…

Reflection

For the Reader

1. Which part of CONNECT feels most familiar to you already?

2. Which part do you feel least confident in—and why?

3. If you imagined a week where "connection came first", what might feel different?

4. What's one thing you could observe or adapt today that might help your child feel seen?

5. What would it mean to approach your role as a caregiver from a place of empowerment, not pressure?

For Professionals: reflecting on practice

▶ How often do I find myself focusing on strategy over clarity?

▶ In what ways could a flexible framework like CONNECT help anchor the families I support?

▶ Do I leave space for parents to build their own insights and voice?

APPENDIX SUGGESTIONS

Appendix A:
The CONNECT Framework Summary
A reminder of the essential tenets.

Appendix K:
Everday CONNECT in Action
Real-life examples across ages and themes.

Chapter Five

Connection First

Why relationship always comes before results

Before we talk about language, routines, or anything else—we start here. **Connection.**

It sounds simple. And it's something most parents instinctively know matters. But in the world of "support", connection often gets crowded out. We become so focused on doing the right things, supporting the right skills, following the right programmes, that we miss the most important thing: the *relationship.*

Children thrive in connection. Not in pressure. Not in performance. Not in endless redirection. When they feel safe, understood, and genuinely *seen*, that's when language blooms. That's when learning happens. That's when the nervous system settles enough for real communication to begin.

More than a buzzword

"Connection" is one of those words that gets thrown around a lot in therapeutic spaces. But when I talk about connection, I don't just mean cuddles and quality time. I mean emotional attunement. Being with your child in a way that says, *I see you. I'm not trying to fix you. I'm here with you, even when things are hard.*

True connection isn't about being calm all the time. It's about being *available*. It's about creating a space where your child doesn't have to mask, perform, or prove.

That kind of connection is the foundation for everything else we'll talk about in this book.

What it looks like in real life

I remember working with a family whose four-year-old daughter had stopped speaking entirely outside the home. Her mum was heartbroken. "She talks to me," she said, "but as soon as we go out, it's like she disappears."

They'd been told to push her—to get her out more, to practise "bravery", to use stickers and praise when she spoke. But it wasn't working. It was just adding pressure.

So we stopped. We pulled back from trying to *get* her to talk. Instead, we focused on helping her feel safe. We created little moments of shared attention—watching bubbles, playing with wind-up toys, reading favourite books in a quiet corner.

Her mum started tuning in more deeply. She let silence hang longer. She smiled instead of prompting. And slowly, her daughter started whispering. Then humming. Then talking—in her own time, in her own way.

Connection first.

Why it's hard

So often, parents are told they need to be "consistent", "in control", and "the authority". But connection asks us to be *responsive*, not rigid. And that can feel scary—especially when behaviour is big, or when progress feels slow.

You might worry that if you focus too much on connection, your child won't learn the skills they need. But here's the truth I've seen time and again:

Connection is not a distraction from learning—it's the doorway to it.

If a child doesn't feel safe, they can't access the part of their brain that allows for flexible thinking, memory, language, or emotional control. Trying to teach a child who doesn't feel connected is like pouring water into a closed bottle.

The work is to open the bottle first.

When connection comes first, communication follows

There's a reason "connection first" comes before even "communication" in the CONNECT Framework. Because communication is the outcome of safety, not the beginning of it.

So many of the children I've worked with didn't start speaking because someone taught them how. They started speaking because someone connected with them deeply enough that they *wanted* to share.

Even the act of noticing a child's body language and responding to it with curiosity can be the beginning of powerful communication. It says: *You don't have to speak for me to understand you. You don't have to prove anything. I'm here, and I'm listening.*

And from that place, words can grow.

What you can do today

You don't need to overhaul your parenting to build connection. You don't need more time, or more toys, or a more perfect version of yourself.

Here's what helps:

► **Be present** in short, focused moments— even five minutes of eye-level play can shift the mood.

- **Be curious** rather than corrective. "I wonder what's tricky right now?" opens far more doors than "Don't do that."

- **Let silence breathe.** You don't have to fill the space with talking. Sometimes your stillness is the invitation.

- **Notice the small wins**—a glance, a giggle, a moment of calm after chaos.

- **Repair when needed.** Connection doesn't mean you never get it wrong. It means you *come back* after rupture, and that's what builds trust.

A note on older children

Connection is just as important with teens. In fact, it might be more important—because the social demands are higher, the mask is tighter, and the world feels louder.

But connection looks different with older kids. It might be sitting quietly next to them while they game. It might be driving without talking until they're ready. It might be holding boundaries while still holding the relationship.

Connection isn't soft. It's **strong.** It's what allows you to show up again and again—even when you're not sure it's making a difference. Because it is.

Reflection

For the Reader

1. When do you feel most connected to your child?

2. What gets in the way of connection right now?

3. Are there moments you've seen your child soften when you slow down?

4. What's one small shift you could make to be more available or present this week?

5. How can you repair after a hard moment, rather than trying to prevent them all?

For Professionals: reflecting on practice

- ▶ How do I currently prioritise connection in my sessions or classroom?

- ▶ What might be getting in the way of connection—for me or the family?

- ▶ Have I unintentionally treated emotional safety as secondary to outcomes?

APPENDIX SUGGESTIONS

Appendix C:
Conversation Starters & Talking Ahead Scripts
This resource supports building everyday connection in day-to-day life.

Appendix F:
Regulation Strategies for Real Life
When connection and co-regulation go hand-in-hand.

Chapter Six

Observe And Adapt

Noticing what matters, changing what helps

We're often told to "watch and wait". But rarely are we told what we're watching for— or how to use what we see to make life better for our child.

That's what this chapter is about.

Because "observe and adapt" isn't just a parenting slogan. It's a mindset. It's the practice of *slowing down enough to notice*, and then *tweaking what we can control* so our child can feel more successful, safe, and seen.

Seeing with softer eyes

We tend to scan for what's not working:

- What's missing from their speech?
- Why aren't they managing that transition?
- What's wrong with how they're behaving?

But observation within the CONNECT Framework isn't about spotting problems—it's about spotting *patterns*. It's about asking:

- ► What's going on beneath that behaviour?
- ► When do they seem most regulated?
- ► What helps them connect?
- ► What's too much, or not enough?

And then, once we've seen something clearly, we gently *adapt*.

Sometimes that means changing the environment. Sometimes it means adjusting expectations. Sometimes it means changing ourselves—how we speak, how we wait, how we move closer or give space.

STORY: Two chairs and a slice of toast

I once worked with a little boy who had meltdowns nearly every morning. His mum described him as "fine until breakfast," and then everything went downhill. She'd tried earlier nights, more protein, less screen time, you name it.

But when we slowed things down, when we observed more closely, we noticed something strange.

He was fine until she moved *his* chair.

Every morning, she'd scoot his chair in while

placing the toast down—an act of care, done without thinking. But for him, it was unpredictable. He didn't like being touched from behind. It triggered dysregulation before the day had even started.

We made one change: she let him scoot his own chair.

That's it.

The meltdowns stopped.

That's the power of *observation and adaptation*. No complex intervention. No behaviour chart. Just noticing and adjusting with empathy.

Why this matters

Many of the families I support feel overwhelmed by the number of things they're "supposed" to be doing:
Visuals. Schedules. Targets. Programmes.

But so often, what shifts things isn't a new tool. It's a new lens. When parents start noticing differently, they start responding differently—and everything softens.

The pressure lifts. The relationship becomes easier. The child feels safer.

That's the shift from *reactive parenting* to *responsive parenting*.

What to observe

Here are just a few things I often invite families to observe—not with judgement, but with curiosity:

- ► **Sensory cues:** Does your child cover their ears, squint, hold their body stiffly, rock, or seek out deep pressure?

- ► **Transitions:** What helps your child move between activities smoothly? What throws them?

- ► **Play:** What toys or games do they return to again and again? What seems to spark joy?

- ► **Language attempts:** Even if they're not speaking, do they gesture, glance, reach, pause, or use facial expressions in a communicative way?

- ► **Regulation patterns:** What times of day are easiest? Hardest? What helps them stay calm?

The goal isn't to build a report. It's to *understand* your child's rhythms better.

What to adapt

Once you've observed something useful, it's time to adapt. This doesn't mean changing everything overnight. It's about small shifts— ones that respect your child's needs and your family's capacity.

Here are examples of small adaptations that have made a big difference:

- ► **Reducing language load:** Using one-step instructions instead of layered speech.
- ► **Prepping before transitions:** Saying "First coat, then car" with visual support.
- ► **Adjusting routines:** Swapping a chaotic morning TV show for quiet music.
- ► **Changing your position:** Sitting side-by-side instead of face-to-face if direct eye contact is overwhelming.
- ► **Making space:** Allowing longer wait times after asking a question or offering a choice.

Take Amira, for example. She was sitting at the kitchen table, shoulders hunched, maths sheet untouched. "I can't do this," she sighed, already withdrawing. Her dad's instinct was to encourage—or insist—that she "just try".

But instead of pressing on, he paused. He noticed her posture, the tension in her voice, and the way she was pulling back from the task. Those cues told him more than the words did.

So he adapted. Sliding the sheet a little closer, he said, "Let's do the first one together. First, we'll try one, then if it feels too much, we'll put the rest aside."

That tiny shift changed everything. With the pressure lowered, Amira attempted one problem, then surprised herself by managing a few more. He wasn't fixing the whole situation; he was showing her she was safe, supported, and not alone—and that was enough for learning to follow.

Sometimes the biggest breakthrough doesn't come from *doing more*, but from *doing less—differently.*

From "fixing" to flow

The magic of "observe and adapt" is that it removes the pressure to *fix*. You don't need to change your child. You just need to notice what's working—and what isn't—and make compassionate changes.

This mindset is especially helpful for children with sensory differences, anxiety, or executive function challenges. If something's hard for your child, it's not because they're *being* difficult. It's because they're *having* difficulty.

And observation helps you see where that difficulty lies.

Adaptation helps you do something about it—without punishment, shame, or overload.

For teens and older children

Observation doesn't stop when your child grows. In fact, it becomes even more important—and more subtle.

A teen who's suddenly silent might be processing something overwhelming. A child who seems withdrawn may be protecting themselves from sensory or social exhaustion. Teens often express distress by *withdrawing*—which is harder to notice than big behaviour.

When we observe with curiosity, we stay in relationship—even when words are few.

Adapting for teens might look like:

- ► Adjusting expectations around mealtimes or social events
- ► Offering new ways to communicate (text, journaling, side-by-side walks)

► Providing recovery time after stressful
   school days

The approach doesn't change. The shape of
it does.

Reflection

For the Reader

1. What's something your child does that you haven't fully understood yet?

2. Can you think of a moment this week that went wrong—and rewind it with curious eyes?

3. When does your child seem most calm and connected? What about that moment might be worth repeating?

4. What small adaptation could you try tomorrow that might ease a tough moment?

5. What helps *you* stay in observation mode, instead of defaulting to correction or control?

For Professionals: reflecting on practice

▶ When do I observe without interrupting?

▶ How might I help caregivers slow down and notice before reacting?

▶ Where could small adaptations replace larger interventions?

APPENDIX SUGGESTIONS

Appendix B:
CONNECT Reflection & Planner Page Templates
This resource supports observational reflection at home and in day-to-day life.

Appendix F:
Regulation Strategies for Real Life
Many adaptations stem from regulatory insight.

Chapter Seven

Natural Routines

Why the everyday is exactly where it happens

Therapy can sometimes feel like a separate world—an hour carved out of real life, in a quiet room with laminated visuals and structured targets. But for most families, that's not where growth happens.

Language, connection, and regulation aren't built in therapy rooms. They're built in *life*.

That's what this chapter is all about. Not creating new tasks or setting up the "perfect" moment. But recognising the incredible power that already exists in the little things you do every single day.

Let's stop trying to "fit it in"

One of the biggest shifts I've seen in families is the moment they stop asking:
"When am I supposed to do all this?"
and start asking:
"Where is it already happening?"

You don't need to find extra time for play-based learning or therapy games. You're already doing *so much* that matters. Breakfast. Getting dressed. Bedtime. Walking to the park. Loading the washing machine. Sitting in the garden.

Every single one of those moments holds potential for communication, regulation, shared joy, and skill-building—*if we can learn to see them through that lens.*

A morning like any other

Let's take a completely typical routine: getting dressed.

This is often one of the hardest parts of the day. Everyone's tired. Time is tight. And children often resist—especially if there are sensory challenges, communication breakdowns, or simply too many steps to process.

Now, let's shift the lens:

- ► **Connection:** Can I greet my child with warmth instead of rushing in with a list of tasks?

- ► **Observe and adapt:** Are there certain clothes that trigger overwhelm? Can we prep an outfit the night before or offer a simple choice?

- ► **Natural routines:** This is already happening—so how can I embed simple language into it?

→ *"Socks on. One sock... two socks!"*

→ *"First your t-shirt, then your jumper."*

→ *"Where does your arm go? Let's find the sleeve!"*

► **Communication as an outcome of regulation:** Can I pause and co-regulate if dressing becomes stressful? Am I adding language when they're ready— not when they're dysregulated?

It's not about getting through it faster. It's about turning what's already happening into a *moment of connection and learning.*

Breakfast, not worksheets

So often, we focus on language as something that has to be *taught*. But it grows in the breakfast routine just as well as in a structured session.

Pouring cereal? That's sequencing, vocabulary, and turn-taking.

Spilling milk? That's emotional regulation and problem-solving.

Butter on toast? That's requesting, commenting, describing—especially if you slow down and narrate with intention:

> → *"Do you want jam or butter?"*
>
> → *"I'm spreading it slowly... look, all the way to the edge!"*
>
> → *"Oops! Milk splash. Let's wipe it up together."*

The key is to give your child time to think and process what is being said in a real life context. Pausing and holding space encourages thinking and turn taking.

This isn't about doing more. It's about *being present* for what's already there.

Lying in the garden

One of the most powerful moments I had with one of my own children came not during a planned activity but lying on a blanket in the garden.

They were dysregulated. I was tired. We weren't "doing therapy". We were just... there.

We watched the leaves move. I mirrored their humming. I let the silence settle.

And then they whispered something—a sentence, fully formed. Not because I prompted them. But because they felt safe enough to share.

That moment reminded me: *Nature slows us down. Presence opens the door.*

Lying in the garden. Walking to the park. Watching birds at the window. These are *natural routines*, too. They ground us. They invite connection.

And they're completely free.

The bedtime shift

Bedtime can feel like the hardest part of the day. But it also holds beautiful opportunities—when it's not rushed or overloaded with demands.

Think about what's already part of your evening:

◊ The routine of pyjamas, teeth brushing, stories
◊ The rhythm of lights dimming, rooms softening
◊ The closeness of cuddles, the chance to reflect on the day

We can embed connection here, too:

→ *"Let's talk ahead about tomorrow. What's the first thing we'll do?"*

→ *"I loved the way you helped your sister today."*

→ *"What colour was your best moment today?"*

No targets. No pressure. Just a ritual of warmth and safety that builds language through *relationship*.

What natural routines are not

This isn't about turning every routine into a lesson. It's not about turning playtime into therapy. It's not about constant narration or pushing speech.

It's about *slowing down enough* to recognise

that your everyday life is already a rich language and connection environment.

And if something isn't working—if the bedtime routine is always a battle, or the walk to school ends in tears—then it's not about trying harder. It's about observing and gently adapting. Just like in the last chapter.

A PARENT'S STORY: The park as a language playground

One family I supported had a toddler who struggled with transitions and speech clarity. They didn't have time for extra sessions during the week. But they *did* walk to the park every Saturday morning.

We focused on making that routine work for them.

Instead of rushing, they built in space:

- **Talking ahead:** *"First breakfast, then shoes, then park."*
- **Predictable rhythm:** *"Swings first, then roundabout."*
- **Pausing to comment and wait:** *"Wow, you're so high!"*… and then pausing, allowing space for a look, a smile, or a word.

They began to notice so much more—shared attention, gesturing, more spontaneous words.

They didn't need to do *more*. They just needed to *see what was already there*.

Natural doesn't mean effortless

This isn't about making life feel easy. It's about making life feel *real*.

There will still be socks thrown across the room. Melted-down mornings. Tantrums at the toothbrush. That's life with kids. But when you trust that those moments *count*—that they *matter*—something shifts.

You stop seeing them as wasted time and start seeing them as *opportunities to reconnect.*

Reflection

For the Reader

1. Which daily routines feel the most stressful in your home right now?

2. What's one natural routine that already feels like a good moment of connection?

3. Can you name three routines that you do every single day without planning? (e.g. snack time, brushing hair, car journeys)

4. What small shift could make one of those routines feel calmer or more connected?

5. How can you give yourself permission to slow down in just one of those moments this week?

For Professionals: reflecting on practice

- ▶ Do I encourage parents to embed strategies in real life—or to recreate therapy tasks?

- ▶ Am I over-relying on tools, resources or visuals? Could a simpler interaction suffice?

APPENDIX SUGGESTIONS

Appendix B:
CONNECT Reflection & Planner Page Templates
These offer a way for you to plan or record natural routines that you are using.

Appendix C:
Conversation Starters & Talking Ahead Scripts
This resource can help you to embed language in daily routines.

Chapter Eight

Neurodiversity-Affirming Practice

Seeing difference, not deficit

There's a quiet shift that happens when we stop asking, *"How do I fix this?"* and start asking, *"What do they need to flourish?"*

That's the shift at the heart of neurodiversity-affirming practice. It's about recognising that our children aren't broken. They aren't behind. They aren't less-than. They are *wired differently*—and they deserve to be supported in a way that honours who they are.

More than a buzzword

"Neurodiversity-affirming" is a term that's becoming more common, but it's not always clear what it means in real life.

It doesn't mean letting everything go or never supporting your child.
It doesn't mean avoiding structure, boundaries, or goals.
It means this:

We stop trying to make the child fit the system—and start making the system fit the child.

We stop seeing difference as disorder.
We stop pathologizing behaviour that is actually communication.
We stop asking, *"How can I get them to do this like everyone else?"*
And we start asking, *"What do they need in order to feel safe, connected, and able to show us who they are?"*

The moment that changed my view

In the early years of parenting, I sometimes found myself caught between what I knew professionally and what I felt instinctively. Certain experiences didn't match what I'd expected—and the strategies I'd previously relied on didn't always seem to land.

I was emotionally exhausted, unsure how to interpret and respond to what I was seeing. And then my friend reminded me not to view my child through a deficit lens.

That became an anchor. It helped me let go of needing the perfect answer—and instead focus on being present, responsive, and willing to see things through a new lens.

And it's something I now say to almost every parent I work with—and just as often, to the professionals who work with me as a parent too. Because deficit-thinking runs deep in our systems. It's baked into developmental norms, assessments, reports, and even the well-meaning advice we give to families.

But it is *not* the foundation of good support.

Language matters

I no longer say "autism spectrum disorder". Because it's not a disorder that needs curing. It's a neurological difference that needs understanding.

I don't ask, *"What's wrong with this child?"*
I ask, *"What's happening for this child—and how can we support them to thrive?"*

When we shift our language, we shift the emotional tone of the entire conversation. We invite curiosity instead of correction. We create space instead of fear.

Affirming doesn't mean avoiding

There's a misconception that affirming neurodiversity means lowering expectations or never working on anything challenging.

That's not the case.

What it means is that we're not working *against* the child's natural neurology—we're working *with* it. We're not trying to erase their differences or hide their distress. We're helping them *understand* those things. And we're helping parents understand them, too.

For example:

- If a child is overwhelmed in noisy classrooms, we don't "toughen them up". We adjust the sensory environment and teach regulation strategies.

- If a teen doesn't make eye contact, we don't force it. We focus on connection through other means—body language, shared interest, time spent side-by-side.

- ▸ If a child uses scripts or echolalia, we don't rush to extinguish it. We explore how it helps them process, and what they might be trying to communicate through it.

Parenting with this lens

Affirming practice isn't just a clinical stance. It's a parenting posture, too.

It means noticing what your child does when they're most themselves.
It means letting go of what other people think they *should* be doing.
It means celebrating the joyful quirks and patterns that make your child who they are.

It also means being willing to unlearn. To stop measuring progress by someone else's chart. To stop comparing your child to their peers—and instead, to compare them to who they were yesterday, or last month, or last year.

That's the kind of progress that matters.

A shift that frees everyone

I once worked with a teenager who had been described, over and over, as "non-compliant". She was autistic, bright, creative—and completely disengaged from traditional education. Every support plan focused on how to manage her "defiance".

But when I met her, it was clear she wasn't defiant. She was overwhelmed. She was trying to protect herself from environments that didn't make sense to her. She wasn't "non-compliant"—she was *self-protective.*

So we adapted. We reduced language load. We gave her choices. We explained what we were doing *before* we did it. We created space to regulate—without making her feel like a problem.

And she opened up. Not because we "fixed" her—but because we finally stopped trying.

That's what this chapter is about. Seeing clearly. Supporting compassionately. Creating space for our children—and ourselves—to be who we are.

Reflection

For the Reader

1. What language do you find yourself using about your child? Is it deficit-based or difference-based?

2. When does your child seem most regulated, connected, and free to be themselves?

3. Are there any traits or behaviours you've been taught to see as a problem that might actually be a clue to what your child needs?

4. What would it look like to affirm your child's way of being this week?

5. What do _you_ need to feel more confident in challenging deficit narratives?

For Professionals: reflecting on practice

- ▶ How has my experience and understanding of neurodiversity evolved in recent years?

- ▶ Do my reports and sessions reflect a strength-based lens?

- ▶ Where might I still be unconsciously prioritising 'typical' benchmarks?

APPENDIX SUGGESTIONS

Appendix H:
Scripts for Siblings, Grandparents & Extended Support
This resource is designed for supporting others to understand neurodivergence.

Appendix I:
Language for Reports, Forms & Advocacy Documents
This resource is to encourage affirming, accurate phrasing.

Chapter Nine

Empowered Caregivers

You are the expert on your child

So many of the parents I meet come into sessions carrying an invisible weight.

They sit down with me—tired, uncertain, determined—and I can almost feel the pressure coming off them in waves.

They've read the reports. They've Googled at 2am. They've filled in EHCP forms, sat through meetings, held it together during phone calls, and sometimes, cried in the car outside.

And almost every single one of them says a version of the same thing:

"I don't know if I'm doing this right."

But here's the truth I wish every parent could carry with them, always:

You are the expert on your child.
Your voice matters.
And this work doesn't happen without you.

The disconnect we don't talk about

The system—whether health, education, or support services—doesn't always treat parents like experts. It often treats them like passive recipients of information.

But when we do that, we miss the most important thing: parents already hold the map.

You know the rhythms of your child's day.

You know what soothes them, what lights them up, what makes them shut down.

You've seen the patterns no professional has the time to see.

You've lived through the meltdowns and the breakthroughs, and all the silent spaces in between.

It's not uncommon for parents to notice progress before professionals do. Sometimes it's a first word, or a burst of spontaneous language that seems to come from nowhere—but really comes from *safety*. Home is often where pressure is lowest and predictability is highest. That matters.

I previously worked with a family where the parent kept a quiet record of the little phrases her daughter was saying when no one else was listening. She even started recording snippets of audio—not to boast, but to bring proof to a meeting with a Teacher of the Deaf who had gently questioned the child's potential. She told me, *"I just wanted them to believe me. I wasn't making it up."*

She wasn't. Her daughter's progress was real. And it held clues about what helped her thrive.

From self-doubt to self-trust

It's no surprise that parents feel disempowered. When you're handed a long report full of jargon and developmental scores, it's easy to start second-guessing yourself.

I've seen parents in meetings shrink back into themselves—not because they don't care, but because they feel like they don't know enough. Like their instincts don't carry weight.

But what I've also seen—again and again—is the moment that something clicks. When a parent hears me say, *"You already have what you need,"* and they look up, surprised.

It's not just a line. It's a truth.

You are **already** doing more right than you think.

STORY: A mum who found her voice

One parent I worked with had been through years of interventions with her teenage son. At one point, she had been so involved—on every panel, at every meeting, tracking every detail of his EHCP.

But over time, the system had worn her down. The plan was getting watered down. Professionals kept changing. They praised her son's "independence" without recognising how much scaffolding she was still providing every day.

She said to me, *"I feel like I have to convince people he still needs support. Like I'm being difficult."*

But she wasn't being difficult. She was being **clear.** She could see what others couldn't because she lived it. Her son still needed the same understanding and adjustments—just in new ways.

So we worked on how she could speak with strength and softness in meetings. How she could use specific language that professionals would respond to. How she could hold her own ground, without apology.

By the time his next review came, she walked in with clarity, calm, and confidence. And she got the support reinstated.

That's empowerment.
Not becoming louder. Becoming **steadier.**

Why it doesn't always look the same everywhere

Sometimes parents and professionals seem to be describing two different children. *"He never does that at school"* or *"She doesn't show that at home."*

When that happens, it's not a sign that one side is wrong. It's a prompt to get curious. What's different about the environment? The expectations? The transitions, the noise levels, the sense of safety?

If your child is doing something at home that they don't yet do in other settings— it matters. It means that the skill is there. And it's up to all of us to understand what's supporting it.

So if you're a parent seeing progress that others haven't yet seen, don't doubt it. Describe it. Share it. Let's be detectives together—not just measuring what your child can do in one place, but understanding *why* it's working there, and how we can help it grow in other settings too.

Building that confidence

Empowerment doesn't happen overnight. It grows in layers. But here are a few ways I've seen parents begin to build it:

- **Document patterns:** Keep notes of what you notice. They don't have to be polished. Bullet points are enough. You're building a bank of insight.

- **Reflect before reacting:** Give yourself time to think through what your child's behaviour might be telling you, instead of just jumping to strategies.

- **Ask questions:** Professionals should welcome them. If something doesn't make sense, say so. You deserve to understand.

- ► **Advocate gently but firmly:** "This doesn't reflect what we see at home" is a powerful phrase.

- ► **Connect with others:** Hearing *"me too"* from another parent can be a lifeline.

Your child needs you—not perfection

Here's something I want every caregiver to hear clearly: **you don't need to do it all perfectly.**

You don't need an Instagram-worthy routine. You don't need laminated visuals or a colour-coded therapy binder. You don't need to keep up with the parent who seems to be doing it all effortlessly online.

What your child needs most is you—**present, attuned, learning, and showing up in real life, not curated life.**

We are parenting in a culture that whispers—sometimes shouts—that we're not enough. That someone else is doing it better. That if we just tried harder, followed more experts, or bought one more resource, we'd unlock the secret to success.

It's not true. And it's not helping.

This comparison culture can be quietly toxic. It can make us strive for a version of parenting that isn't even real—and in doing so, it pulls us away from the connection that really matters. I've seen parents push themselves to the edge trying to keep up, and in the process, lose sight of the things they were doing *right all along.*

Sometimes the pressure to "get it right" undoes all the good that's already happening.

So, here's your permission to filter. To ignore the advice that doesn't serve you. To mute the noise that makes you question yourself. And to trust that the connection you build with your child in your ordinary moments is already doing so much more than you realise.

Empowered caregiving isn't about getting everything perfect. It's about **being available.** It's about knowing when to pause, when to rest, and when to reach out. And it's about giving yourself grace on the hard days—not guilt.

We'll talk more about this in Chapter Eleven. And we'll explore it even more deeply in **Book Two: Connected Parent**, where we dig into how identity, expectations, and family culture shape the way we parent.

But for now, just know this:

You don't need to be perfect.
You just need to be real.
And your child already knows the difference.

A note for the professionals

Please know that when you speak with a parent, you're not just delivering information. You're shaping their sense of whether or not they're capable—and how welcome their insights are in the process of support.

There may be times when a parent shares something you haven't seen yourself. Maybe it's a skill the child shows at home, a behaviour that hasn't appeared in school, or a moment of progress that feels unexpected.

When that happens, it doesn't mean someone is wrong. It simply means there's more to discover.

In my experience, these moments are rich with potential. They can give us clues about what's supporting that child's success—clues we might miss if we only focus on what we've personally observed.

We might ask:

- ▶ *"What's helping this happen at home?"*
- ▶ *"Is there something about the environment, the rhythm, or the relationship that we can learn from?"*
- ▶ *"How could we use that understanding to bridge the gap between settings?"*

This kind of reflection isn't about blame—it's about building trust. It's about recognising that every adult in the child's life holds a piece of the puzzle. And when we take the time to piece those perspectives together, our support becomes stronger, not softer.

So, if a parent sees something you haven't yet seen, perhaps the question isn't *"Is that really happening?"* but *"What can we learn from the fact that it is?"*

Because when we honour what families notice—and what children show us in the safety of those relationships—we make space for progress to grow across every part of their world.

And when we empower caregivers, we empower children.

Reflection

For the Reader

1. When was the last time you trusted your instinct as a parent—and it turned out to be right?

2. Have there been times when you felt shut down in a meeting or conversation about your child?

3. What would help you feel more confident or calm in those moments?

4. What strengths do you bring to your child's life that no one else can?

5. If you believed, even for today, that *you are the expert on your child*, how might that shift your choices?

For Professionals: reflecting on practice

▶ Do I actively name and reflect the parent's expertise in sessions?

▶ How might I shift from instructing to partnering?

▶ Have I ever downplayed a caregiver's insight without meaning to?

APPENDIX SUGGESTIONS

Appendix D:
School and Professional Advocacy Guide
Your companion in those daunting meetings!

Appendix I:
Language for Reports, Forms & Advocacy Documents
This resource is to encourage affirming, accurate phrasing.

Chapter Ten

Communication as an Outcome of Regulation (and Connection)

Why safety and connection come first

Communication is often seen as the *goal*. But in the CONNECT Framework, it's the outcome. Not the first priority—but the natural result of everything that comes before it.

That one shift changes everything.

Because when we stop focusing on *getting our child to talk or making them answer*, and start focusing on what their nervous system needs, we unlock something far more powerful than words.

We create the conditions for connection.

What if it's not about talking?

Let me say something that surprises many families the first time they hear it:

If your child is dysregulated, they cannot access meaningful communication.

It doesn't matter how bright they are. It doesn't matter how strong their vocabulary is. When a child is in fight, flight, freeze—or even just low-level overwhelm—they can't fully listen, process, sequence, or express themselves clearly.

Their nervous system isn't designed to multitask between *survival* and *speech*.

So if we push for more words or faster answers in those moments, we're not helping them communicate—we're asking them to do the impossible.

What's really going on?

Here's what regulation might look like in everyday life:

◊   A toddler hiding under the table before nursery.

◊   A child clenching their jaw, stiffening their shoulders, or turning away.

◊   A teen going completely silent or saying "I don't care" to everything.

◊   A child laughing at inappropriate times or zoning out during conversations.

None of these are signs of defiance. They're signals.

When we see behaviour through the lens of regulation, everything starts to make more sense. We don't need to label or punish—we need to *support*.

And when we support regulation, communication becomes possible again.

The story of a shift

One little boy I worked with had huge outbursts during transitions. His language seemed to disappear the moment he was asked to stop one thing and start another.

His mum kept saying, *"He knows what to do. He just won't do it."*

But what we discovered together was this: the outbursts weren't about disobedience.

They were about dysregulation. He was overwhelmed, and his brain was in a state of threat.

So, we shifted the focus.

We stopped saying, *"Use your words"*, and started supporting co-regulation first. We brought in calming strategies, built in pauses, softened our voice tone, and gave space. We talked ahead. We gave him language *after* the regulation had returned—not before.

And guess what?

He started using words again. He asked for help. He explained what he didn't like. He even started suggesting his own strategies.

His communication hadn't been lost—it had just been hidden under stress.

Co-regulation is the bridge

We talk a lot about self-regulation. But it doesn't come out of nowhere. Children learn to self-regulate *through* co-regulation.

That means having a calm adult nearby who:

- ► Sees the struggle without judgment
- ► Holds the emotional space without rushing in to fix
- ► Models breathing, softening, and waiting
- ► Reassures, *"I've got you"*, even when things feel messy.

This isn't about staying calm in a robotic way. It's about staying *connected*—even when your child isn't able to meet you there yet.

When a child learns that they don't have to *be okay* to be loved, they begin to feel safe. And that safety is where communication starts to grow again.

Regulation before strategy

Many well-meaning interventions jump straight into strategies:

— *"Ask for help."*

— *"Use your calm-down card."*

— *"Say how you feel."*

But those only work if the child is regulated enough to access them.

We need to lay the groundwork first:

► What helps your child *return to regulation?*

► What's their sensory profile telling you?

► What routines or environments help them feel safe?

► What's your own nervous system doing when theirs starts to spiral?

If a strategy isn't working, the problem might not be the strategy. It might be that regulation hasn't been prioritised first.

Let's redefine progress

Progress isn't just longer sentences or clearer speech. It's:

- ✓ A child staying at the table for two extra minutes.
- ✓ A teen saying *"I need a break"* instead of storming off.
- ✓ A meltdown that lasts 15 minutes instead of 45.
- ✓ A look, a nod, a glance toward the thing they want to say.

These are signs that the nervous system is softening. That the connection is safe. That the scaffolding is holding.

And that's the foundation for all the communication skills that follow.

A note for families of non-speaking children

If your child is non-speaking or minimally verbal, this chapter is especially for you.

Because the pressure to *"get them talking"* can be relentless. And sometimes, it makes everyone feel like they're failing.

But please hear this:

Communication is so much bigger than speech.
And regulation is the key that unlocks all of it.

When we slow down, attune, and co-regulate, we create space for alternative communication to emerge—gestures, glances, vocalisations, AAC, sign language, or shared moments of joy.

You are not behind. You are building the conditions for something deeper than words.

Reflection

For the Reader

1. When is your child most regulated? What helps that happen?

2. What signs of dysregulation do you tend to notice first?

3. Are there times when you've tried to prompt communication—but your child was actually in a stress state?

4. How could you prioritise co-regulation this week, even for a few minutes a day?

5. What's one sign of progress that might be easy to miss—but is still deeply meaningful?

For Professionals: reflecting on practice

▶ Do I pause to consider regulation before prompting language?

▶ What signs of dysregulation am I attuned to—and which might I be missing?

▶ How can I better support co-regulation, even when time is tight?

APPENDIX SUGGESTIONS

Appendix F:
Regulation Strategies for Real Life
Key to this chapter's central message.

Appendix G:
Supporting Non-Speaking Communicators
This resource directly complements this chapter's final section.

Chapter Eleven

Togetherness

You're not meant to do this alone

At the heart of everything in the CONNECT Framework is this quiet but radical truth:

You were never meant to do this alone.

Not the parenting.
Not the therapy.
Not the wondering at night, the advocating in meetings, the interpreting of behaviour that no one else seems to understand.

Togetherness doesn't mean perfect harmony. It doesn't mean agreeing on everything. It doesn't even mean constant presence. It means belonging. Being part of something bigger than yourself. Being held when things feel heavy—and offering your strength when someone else needs it too.

But what if you *are* doing it alone?

Not everyone has a co-parent. Not everyone has grandparents to help, or a neighbour who offers the school run. Some parents are navigating this journey solo—logistically, emotionally, or both.

And even within two-parent households, it's often the case that one person feels the weight of it more than the other. The lion's share of advocacy, of appointments, of thinking five steps ahead.

So, let's be clear: when I say, *"You're not meant to do this alone"*, I don't mean you need a perfect support network already in place. I mean you deserve one. I mean it's okay to need one. And I mean that your strength isn't defined by how much you carry—it's defined by your willingness to reach out when it's all too much.

Togetherness isn't just about partnership. It's about *relationship*. With others. With your child. With yourself.

We heal in relationship

Children don't develop in isolation—and neither do adults.

The child learning to regulate is doing so in relationship with a caregiver who is holding them.

The parent learning to trust their instincts is doing so in relationship with professionals who see them.

The teacher learning to adapt is doing so in relationship with the family who shows them what matters most.

Progress, growth, repair—all of it happens in the space between people.

So, if you're struggling, stuck, or uncertain… it doesn't mean you're failing. It means you're human. It means your nervous system is stretched thin. It means you need support.

And asking for support doesn't make you weak. It makes you resilient.

True mental resilience isn't about getting everything right or staying calm all the time. It's about **how we recover.** How we respond after a hard morning or a moment we wish we'd handled differently. It's about being able to say, *"That was too much"*, and still keep going.

Resilience doesn't mean silence or self-sufficiency. It means giving yourself permission to be a learning parent.

Therapy doesn't happen in a vacuum

Therapy—at its best—isn't something done *to* a child. It's something that happens *with* the child and their most trusted people. That's why togetherness is built into every fibre of the CONNECT Framework.

We don't hand over a worksheet and send the parent out.
We don't ask the child to perform while the caregiver waits outside.
We work together—even when the roles aren't symmetrical.

Sometimes the parent leads.
Sometimes the therapist guides.

Sometimes the child shows us what's possible in the spaces between.

But the process is always relational. It's *with*, not *for* or *to*.

A moment between two mums

I once facilitated a small group for parents of neurodivergent children. During one of the sessions, a mother was talking about how hard the school run had become. The refusals, the screaming, the judgement from other parents.

Her voice cracked. She said, *"I just want one day when I don't feel like I'm the only one."*

And another mum—quiet until then—reached across the space between them and said, *"You're not. I had the exact same morning."*

There was nothing technical in that exchange. No strategy. No coaching.

Just togetherness. And it changed everything.

That one sentence—*"You're not the only one"*—can be a lifeline. Especially for those parenting without a co-parent, or without family support, or without anyone else in their real-life world who *gets it.*

Sometimes the most important therapeutic tool we can offer is simply being there.

Togetherness doesn't mean closeness all the time

In families, togetherness shows up in lots of different forms:

- ✓ Sitting side-by-side watching TV
- ✓ Preparing snacks in quiet companionship

✓ Being nearby without asking for anything

✓ Checking in with a nod or a squeeze of the hand.

Sometimes we confuse "together" with "talking" or "doing" or "fixing".

But some of the most connected moments I've seen happen in silence. In simply being with each other. In letting the child take the lead. In choosing presence over pressure.

This applies to parenting ourselves too. Sometimes showing up for yourself means **naming that you're overstimulated.** That you're buffering like a loading screen. That you need silence, or space, or snacks.

That isn't selfish. That's modelling emotional fluency and building co-regulation from the inside out.

Shared understanding within families

Togetherness also means supporting the people who share your child's life—siblings, grandparents, partners, family friends.

It's about helping them understand:

- ► Why your child might need certain accommodations
- ► How you're approaching things differently now
- ► That neurodiversity isn't a tragedy—it's part of what makes your child beautifully, uniquely themselves.

But let's not pretend that's always easy.

Some family members might refuse to acknowledge that your child has additional needs. They may dismiss your concerns, ignore your boundaries, or even undermine the work you're doing.

This can be one of the loneliest kinds of loneliness: being surrounded by people who still don't see your child the way you do.

So let's be clear: you are not responsible for convincing everyone. You don't have to manage everyone else's emotions.

You only need to stay grounded in your journey. And if that journey feels shaky right now, let others help you navigate it. Let it evolve through aligned community, not reaction or constant defence.

The double-edged sword of social media

Sometimes, the only place a parent finds people who "get it" is online. A late-night reel. A caption that speaks your reality. A post that makes you say, *"Yes—this."*

These spaces can be lifelines. They can be full of hope, humour, and solidarity.

But they can also be performative, pressurising, and exhausting.

Because social media doesn't show the whole picture. It shows curated versions—perfectly lit snippets of parenting where everyone is smiling and no one is overstimulated or scrubbing blueberries off the ceiling.

And if you're parenting in survival mode, those images can hurt.

So, hold this close: *You don't have to do it perfectly to be doing it well.*

Your child doesn't need curating. They need connection.

The power of community

No one understands the journey of raising a neurodivergent child quite like someone else who's walking it too.

If you're able to connect with other parents—online, in person, in informal ways—it can be life-changing. Not because you'll always get answers, but because you'll get companionship.

That's why spaces like **The CONNECT Parents Circle** exist—not to create a hierarchy of who's doing it "right", but to offer a place where you can show up tired, messy, proud, or confused, and still be met with understanding.

Togetherness is a practice.
It doesn't always come easy.
But it makes everything else more possible.

Professionals need togetherness too

As a therapist, I've learned this the hard way. Trying to carry families, manage paperwork, juggle systems, and hold emotional space can leave professionals isolated too.

We're not exempt from the need for connection.

The best therapy I've ever delivered has always happened in a relational web—with wise colleagues, generous mentors, and families who trusted me enough to let me walk beside them.

We don't need more lone wolves in this work. We need networks.

No more lone wolves

If there's one thing I want you to carry from this chapter, it's this:

You are not supposed to carry it all.
Not in your home.
Not in your school.
Not in your appointments.
Not in your heart.

Whether you have a partner or not.
Whether your family is helpful or not.
Whether you have three friends or none right now.

You deserve togetherness.

Togetherness is what keeps us steady. It's what allows us to rest. It's what creates the kind of safety that lets communication bloom—not just for children, but for parents too.

Reflection

For Professionals: reflecting on practice

▶ How do I contribute to the sense of 'team' around a child?

▶ What small action could I take to help a family feel less alone?

▶ Where might I need more connection and support in my own professional role?

APPENDIX SUGGESTIONS

Appendix E:
Recommended Resources
Community-building and seeking further support.

Appendix H:
Scripts for Siblings, Grandparents & Extended Support
Designed to support shared understanding.

For the Reader

1. **Who helps you feel less alone—even if they're not physically with you?** This might be a person, a message, a group, or even a sentence you return to.

2. **Where in your life do you carry more than your fair share—and what would it mean to set that down, even for a moment?**

3. **What does togetherness look like in your home, especially during hard moments?** Is it a glance, a pause, a shared breath, or stepping outside together?

4. **When you feel overstimulated or on the edge, how do you recognise it—and what helps you recover?**

5. **How do you care for your own nervous system, not just your child's?** What could support look like if it were built for you, too?

6. **If you could share one truth about your child—or your parenting—with someone who doesn't yet understand, what would you want them to hear?**

Chapter Twelve

The **CONNECT** Framework at a Glance

A return to what matters most

You've travelled through the heart of the CONNECT Framework—not as a checklist or a programme, but as a way of being. A way of seeing your child with clearer eyes, responding with compassion, and finding strength in your everyday rhythms.

This chapter brings all seven elements together in one place—a simple, reassuring reminder of the threads that hold everything together.

Keep it bookmarked. Come back to it when you're tired or stuck. Let it remind you that even when things feel hard, *you already have the tools you need.*

C Connection First

Everything starts with relationship.
Before goals, before progress, before words—connection is the foundation.
Be with your child, not just around them.
Soften. Slow down. Tune in.
Because when connection is safe, communication becomes possible.

Ask yourself: "How can I show up with presence before pressure?"

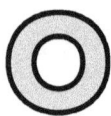

O Observe and Adapt

Notice first. React second.
Your child is constantly communicating through behaviour, movement, tone, and rhythm.
When you observe with curiosity and adapt with care, you become the expert guide they need.

Ask yourself: "What might help this feel easier for both of us?"

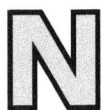

N Natural Routines

You don't need to carve out extra time.
Your daily life is already filled with opportunities—putting on shoes, brushing teeth, sharing toast.

Language lives in these moments. So does connection. So does confidence.

Ask yourself: "Where is the opportunity hiding in what we already do?"

N Neurodiversity-Affirming Practice

Your child isn't broken.
Their brain is wired differently—and that difference is real, valid, and worth honouring. We support them best when we stop trying to "fix" and start asking, "What do they need to flourish?"

Ask yourself: "Am I seeing my child through a lens of deficit or difference?"

E Empowered Caregivers

You are the expert on your child.
You might not always feel it, but your lived experience matters more than any report. When you trust your instincts and share your insight, you lead the way.

Ask yourself: "What do I know about my child that no one else sees?"

C Communication as an Outcome of Regulation

Communication doesn't happen in chaos. It grows when the nervous system feels safe—when a child is regulated, supported, and seen.
If your child can't speak, respond, or engage, the answer isn't to push harder. It's to regulate first.

Ask yourself: "What might their nervous system be telling me right now?"

T Togetherness

You were never meant to do this alone. Togetherness isn't just about support—it's about belonging, even when it looks different to what you imagined.

Progress happens in relationship. Healing happens in relationship.

We grow when we're held—and when we learn how to hold ourselves with gentleness, too.

Ask yourself: "Who is walking this with me—or who could be, if I let them in?"

Final thoughts

The CONNECT Framework isn't something you "do"—it's something you *live.*

It gives you a way to return, again and again, to what matters most:

- **You don't need perfection. You need presence.**
- **You don't need a programme. You need partnership.**
- **You don't need to be everything. You just need to be with them.**

In the final chapter, I'll share some of what I've learned on this journey—not just as a therapist, but as a parent still finding her way.

Chapter Thirteen

What I Know Now

Lessons from the inside out

When I first began this journey—as a young speech and language therapist, full of energy and training—I thought success looked like clarity. Like confidence. Like having the answers.

Now, after years of sitting with families, standing in EHCP reviews, pacing the kitchen floor with worry, holding my own children through tears and happiness and growth...

Success looks different.

It looks like **understanding.**
It looks like **presence.**
It looks like **compassion,** even when the plan goes out the window.
And most of all—it looks like **connection.**

I've learned that progress isn't linear

Children don't develop in neat, upward graphs.
They leap. They plateau. They regress. They surprise you.
Sometimes you spend weeks on one small thing… then they do it when you least expect it.

And the same is true for us as caregivers.

Some days we're calm and patient and present. Other days we're short-tempered, overwhelmed, and trying not to cry at the sight of an uneaten meal.

That's okay. That's real.

I no longer believe in "consistency at all costs". I believe in *repair.* In returning. In showing up again—even when yesterday didn't go how we hoped.

I've learned that instinct is a form of expertise

For a long time, I second-guessed myself. I leaned on protocols and checklists and waited for professionals to validate what I sensed deep down.

But my journey taught me something no training ever could:

I already knew my child. I just needed to trust that knowledge.

Now I tell other parents the same thing: *you are not making it up.*

You're noticing something real.
Your insight has weight.
Your love is diagnostic.

I've learned that slowness isn't a lack of ambition

There's a lot of pressure to keep moving.
Keep progressing. Keep intervening. Keep
checking things off.

But some of the most powerful moments in
my parenting journey—and in my therapy
work—have come in stillness. In slowness. In
stepping back.

When we slow down, we can actually *see*
what's working. We notice the spark in their
eyes, the softness in their shoulders, the way
they return to a favourite game or sound. We
tune in.

And from that quiet space, communication begins to grow again.

I've learned that you don't need to know it all

You don't need to master every strategy.
You don't need to read every book.
You don't need to predict every outcome.

You need to be **anchored** in something that holds you steady.

That's what CONNECT became for me. Not a system to follow, but a set of values to return to. A compass in the messy middle.

And I hope, through this book, it has become a compass for you too.

I've learned that the hard days don't mean you're getting it wrong

The meltdowns, the regressions, the appointments that leave you deflated, the endless forms that make you feel like a number not a name...

Those days don't mean you're not doing enough.

They mean the journey is real.

They mean you're showing up.
They mean your child is doing something brave.
They mean the system might still need changing—but *you* don't need fixing.

I've learned that stories matter

That's why I wrote this book. Not to give you a programme or a polished version of parenting. But to walk alongside you. To say: *You are not alone. It doesn't have to be perfect to be powerful.*

Your story—however messy, quiet, unconventional, or still unfolding—is valid.

It's enough.

And it's one that deserves to be heard.

Final Reflection

For the Reader

1. What have you learned about your child through this journey?

2. What have you learned about yourself?

3. What would you tell your past self, the one who was just starting to notice something different?

4. Which part of the CONNECT Framework will you return to first?

5. What would it mean to believe—today— that you are already enough?

A Letter to You, the Parent Reading This

Dear Parent,

If you've made it to the end of this book, then you've already done something powerful:
You've paused to reflect. You've chosen to explore—not how to fix your child, but how to understand them more deeply, and support them more meaningfully.

That matters.

The day-to-day reality of parenting—especially when your child processes the world differently—can be complex, exhausting, and full of contradictions. Some days you feel like you're holding it all together. Other days, it all feels too much.

That doesn't mean you're doing it wrong. It means you're human.

There's no one right way to parent. But there are ways that feel more aligned. More connected. More respectful of who your child is—and of who you are too.

That's what the CONNECT Framework offers. Not a checklist. Not a set of strategies to apply blindly. But a way to anchor yourself when things are messy, unpredictable, or unclear.

You know your child better than anyone.
Your observations matter.
Your advocacy matters.
Your relationship is not a side note—it's the foundation.

You don't need to do more. You don't need to work harder. You don't need to become someone else. You just need to come back to what you already know and give yourself the permission to lead from that place.

And if you feel unsure, disconnected, or out of your depth?
That's normal.
You're not behind. You're in the middle of a real, evolving process.
And you're not alone.
Keep going. You're already doing more right than you realise.

With warmth,

Susannah

So... What's next?

If this book has spoken to you—if you've found something here that made you pause, feel seen, or shift how you connect with your child—please know this is only the beginning. You don't have to go back to doing it all alone. You're part of something now.

Stay Connected

For weekly insights, real-life tips, and reflections from my ongoing therapy practice, you can follow me on social media:

@Connect_Communication_Therapy

The CONNECT Parent Circle

For those looking to continue the journey in a more personal, supportive space, you're warmly invited to join **The CONNECT Parents Circle**—a private Facebook group where families share, ask, encourage, and connect. You don't need to be an expert—just a human being doing their best.

Together, we're shifting the story. From pressure to presence. From fixing to understanding. From doing more to noticing what's already there.

Coming soon:

Connected Parent

Book Two, **Connected Parent**, is currently in development. It will build on the principles shared in this book but focus even more deeply on **day-to-day messy family life**—how we show up, repair, advocate, and grow alongside our children over time while navigating a world of social media and shifting goals. Whether you're parenting toddlers, teens, or anyone in between, it's for you.

Coming soon:

Online Training & Support

I'm in the process of building a dedicated **training platform**, designed to support families and professionals who want to deepen their understanding of the CONNECT Framework. The platform will include courses, toolkits, and video content to guide and support you— wherever you are in your journey.

www.connectcommunicationtherapy.com

APPENDIX A

The CONNECT Framework® Summary

Real-life communication support starts when we CONNECT.

C - Connection First

💡 **Key Idea:** Before we can expect communication, we need connection.

📋 **Try This:** Prioritise time where nothing is expected—just being together.

EG **Example:** Cuddle on the sofa, sit beside them on the floor, or play side-by-side with no questions or demands.

O - Observe & Adapt

💡 **Key Idea:** Children show us what they need—if we pause and watch.

📋 **Try This:** Step back. Watch quietly for 30 seconds before joining in.

EG **Example:** You notice your child is flapping or pacing. Instead of stopping it, match their energy and join their rhythm first.

N - Natural Routines

Key Idea: Real language happens in real life. No special activities needed.

Try This: Use everyday routines—meals, bath time, getting dressed—as your speech and language sessions.

Example: *"Water on... splash! Let's wash your toes!"* during bath time, building rhythm and shared fun.

N - Neurodiversity-Affirming Practice

Key Idea: Your child doesn't need to be changed—they need to feel safe being themselves.

Try This: Say what you *see* and validate their experience.

Example: *"That tag feels itchy, huh?"* instead of *"Just ignore it."* Honour their sensory world.

E - Empowered Caregivers

💡 **Key Idea:** You don't need to be a therapist—you just need to be *you*, supported.

[TRY THIS] **Try This:** Reflect on what already works in your family and do more of it.

[EG] **Example:** If singing helps with transitions, make it your go-to. *"Time to tidy, tidy away..."* (to the tune of a favourite song).

C - Communication as an Outcome of Regulation

💡 **Key Idea:** Children communicate when they feel safe, seen, and regulated.

[TRY THIS] **Try This:** Co-regulate first—then listen for the communication that follows.

[EG] **Example:** If your child is melting down, sit nearby, breathe deeply, and wait. Once calm returns, the words will come.

T - Togetherness

Key Idea: Learning happens best when we feel held by the people around us — reminded that we're not meant to do this alone.

Try This: Notice who steadies you and whom you naturally lean towards. Let connection be mutual, warm, and real.

Example: Ask yourself, *"Who is walking this with me — and am I letting them in?"*

. . . .

Contact me via my website to request a free printable download of this CONNECT Framework Summary!

www.connectcommunicationtherapy.com

Stick this on the fridge, use it in your setting, or share it with someone who supports your child.

Let it remind you: Connection isn't just part of the process—it *is* the process.

APPENDIX B

CONNECT Reflection & Planner Page Templates

· ·

Why reflection matters

Parents often notice things professionals don't — the small moments of progress, connection, or change that happen in everyday life. But those insights can easily slip away unless we pause to capture them. These pages are a space to slow down, notice, and build on what's working.

Bringing the CONNECT Framework into everyday life

The CONNECT Reflection & Planner pages are designed to help you turn the ideas in this book into lived experiences. Use them alongside each chapter, at the end of a week, or whenever you want to take stock of how things are feeling at home.
There's no right or wrong way to use them — just space for gentle noticing, practical reflection, and small steps forward.

No pressure. No perfection. Just connection.

Weekly Reflection Template

WEEK OF ....

1. What have I noticed this week?

(Any changes, challenges, moments of joy, or patterns in my child's communication or connection)

✎ ....

....

....

....

2. What supported connection this week?

(Think about routines, sensory moments, small wins, or co-regulation)

✎ ....

....

....

....

3. What felt difficult or dysregulating?

✎ ....

....

....

....

4. When did I feel most in sync with my child?

✎ ....

....

....

....

5. What's one small thing I could try or adjust next week?

✎ ....

....

....

....

Goal-Setting or Observation Notes

➤ Short-term focus

(e.g. more shared routines, supporting transitions, modelling language)

....

....

....

....

✓ Why this matters right now

....

....

....

....

? How will I know it's helping?

....

....

....

....

Your Week Through the CONNECT Lens

☐ **Natural routines this week**

Where have communication or shared moments naturally happened? (e.g. bath time, breakfast, walking the dog)

✍ ....

....

....

....

....

☐ **What we're observing**

What are you noticing about your child's cues, moods, interests, or needs this week?

✍ ....

....

....

....

....

Your Week Through the CONNECT Lens (cont.)

☐ **A small adaptation**

One gentle shift we tried or plan to try—
something that meets our child where they
are

✍ ....

....

....

....

....

☐ **Regulation focus**

What supported calm and co-regulation
this week? (e.g. quiet play, movement,
sensory input)

✍ ....

....

....

....

....

Connection moment

A moment we felt in sync, close, or emotionally connected—however small

....

....

....

....

....

Advocacy win or concern

Something we voiced (or want to voice) with others—school, family, professionals

....

....

....

....

....

Daily Snapshot (optional planner)

Day	One thing that felt connected	One challenge I want to reflect on	One small win
M			
T			
W			
T			
F			
S			
S			

☺ **Tip: These notes don't need to be perfect or complete—just truthful.**

✐ **Use bullet points, scribbles, or reflections.**

♥ **Keep it gentle. Keep it real.**

Feel free to recreate these planner pages yourself.

Alternatively, you can use the guided planner pages in my **CONNECT Companion Journal for Families**, which I have developed to accompany you on your CONNECT journey.

APPENDIX C

Conversation Starters & Talking Ahead Scripts

Because what we say—and how we say it—matters.

Transitions & Routines

Use "First... then..." language to make transitions clear and predictable. Keep it visual or action-based when needed.

Script Examples:

→ *"First snack, then coat."*

→ *"First tidy toys, then park."*

→ *"First five more jumps, then stop."*

→ *"First we wait, then we go in."*

For toddlers or early language users:

Keep it short and use gesture or objects: hold the snack and say, *"Snack... then coat"* while pointing.

For older children:

Give more information, invite choice:

→ *"First you finish this level, then it's time to pause and eat. Do you want to set a timer or have a five-minute warning?"*

Co-Regulation & Emotional Moments

These scripts help model emotional language and create safety in dysregulating moments.

Script Examples:

→ *"I can see you're finding this tricky— let's pause together."*

→ *"You're showing me you need space. I'm right here when you're ready."*

→ *"It's okay to feel upset. We can breathe together."*

→ *"That noise was too much, huh? Let's find quiet."*

For toddlers or non-speaking children: Use tone, facial expression, and co-regulation strategies (e.g. humming, rocking, holding hands).

→ *"Breathe with me... in... and out... good."* [whispered gently, rhythmic tone]

For older children:

Normalise feelings and offer regulation options:

→ *"Big feelings aren't bad feelings. Do you want to stomp it out, draw, or sit quietly?"*

Advocacy & Self-Awareness

Support children to understand and advocate for their needs—even if they can't yet say them independently.

Script Examples:

→ *"You can say, 'That's too loud for me.' Or show me with your hands."*

→ *"We can tell your teacher, 'I need a break when it gets busy.'"*

→ *"Your body is telling us it's time to move. That's okay."*

→ *"Let's practice what you want to say if it feels too hard."*

For toddlers or non-speaking children:
Model language paired with gesture or visual card:

→ *"Too loud"* + cover ears

→ *"All done"* + hand signal

For older children or teens:

Support scripting and confidence-building:

→ *"You could say, 'I'm okay, I just need a minute.' Want to try it with me first?"*

Additional Everyday Talking Ahead Examples

Why Talking Ahead Matters

Children often feel safest when they know what's coming next. A simple "First... then..." structure reduces uncertainty, supports regulation, and makes everyday life more predictable. This isn't about rigid schedules— it's about offering a sense of security through language.

Script Examples:

Morning Routine

→ "First pyjamas off... then get dressed."

→ "First toast... then fruit."

Transitions

→ "First coat on... then car."

→ "First shoes... then garden."

💬 **<u>Mealtimes</u>**

→ *"First tidy toys... then lunch."*

→ *"First eat... then pudding."*

💬 **<u>Play</u>**

→ *"First one more turn... then finish game."*

→ *"First pack away bricks... then choose a story."*

💬 **<u>Bedtime</u>**

→ *"First bath... then pyjamas."*

→ *"First teeth... then story."*

General Tips for All Ages

- Keep sentences short and clear, with the key word at the end (acoustic highlighting).

- Match your tone to the regulation level you are working toawards—calm, slow, and warm.

- Use pauses generously. Pauses allow thinking time and act as an invitation to take a turn.

- Respect communication in all forms (gestures, signs, facial expression, AAC).

- Use visuals where possible—objects, pictures, gestures.

- Follow through consistently so your child learns to trust the "then."

- Flex when needed. If your child is dysregulated, pause until they are ready.

Reflection Prompt

Think about a tricky moment in your daily routine:

? How could a simple "First... then..." Talking Ahead script ease that transition?

? Could adding a visual (object, picture, or gesture) make it even clearer?

. . . .

Remember: Your words don't need to be perfect. They need to feel safe.

Talking ahead is about creating clarity, reducing uncertainty, and helping your child feel seen and supported.

APPENDIX D

School & Professional Advocacy Guide

Communicating with confidence—while staying true to what matters most.

. . . .

Why this matters

As a parent or caregiver, you are the expert in your child's regulation, rhythms, and real-world communication. Whether you're at an EHCP/IEP meeting, a school transition, or a review with professionals, this guide offers gentle but firm ways to express what you know helps your child thrive. These pages are a space to slow down, notice, and build on what's working.

. . . .

The CONNECT-Friendly Advocacy Template

You can use this to shape emails, meetings, or reports. Adjust it to suit your tone.

"We're working with a relationship-first framework called the CONNECT approach. It's based on:

— Connection first

— Observation and adaptation

— Natural routines as learning opportunities

— Neurodiversity-affirming practice

— Empowering caregivers and listening to lived experience

— Seeing communication as something that grows out of regulation and connection

— And prioritising togetherness—not top-down training.

— This is what we're using at home, and we'd really value school support that reflects these same values."

Sentence Starters for Advocacy Conversations

✅ **When sharing what's working at home:**

→ "Here's what we're focusing on at home right now: _____."

→ "What really helps my child stay regulated is _____."

→ "Our best communication happens during _____, like bath time or school pick-up chats."

→ "We've found that co-regulation is the first step to any kind of communication."

✓ **When requesting support that aligns with CONNECT:**

→ "Our approach is relationship-first—we'd like support that reflects that."

→ "We'd love school to notice and respond to *what's underneath* a behaviour, not just what it looks like."

→ "Instead of extra requests or compliance goals, we're focusing on safety, shared routines, and confidence."

→ "Could we create a consistent 'safe adult' relationship for my child at school to build trust over time?"

Sentence Starters for Advocacy Conversations (cont.)

✓ **When attending a meeting (EHCP, IEP, or other target review):**

→ "Before we talk targets, can we start with what's going well and what helps my child feel safe?"

→ "I'd like to bring in what's working at home so we can build on it together."

→ "Can we look at how my child is being supported to regulate and co-regulate in the school environment?"

→ "Could we frame communication as something that emerges from connection, rather than a checklist of spoken goals?"

✅ **When talking about sensory needs or emotional regulation:**

→ "My child's body tells us a lot—
sometimes more than their words do."

→ "They're not being difficult; they're
telling us it's *too difficult.*"

→ "We're learning that what looks like
refusal is often overwhelm."

→ "Sensory breaks, quiet transitions,
or just time with a trusted adult are
regulation tools, not rewards."

Sentence Starters for Advocacy Conversations (cont.)

✓ **Closing the loop - suggested language for joint planning:**

→ "Let's keep checking in about what's working—we're all learning together."

→ "If something's not working in school, let's find the 'why' underneath it."

→ "Could we agree to try this for a few weeks and reflect on what we notice?"

→ "Can we make space for ongoing communication between home and school—not just during reviews?"

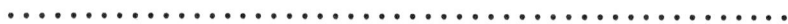

Remember: You don't need to justify your approach.

You're bringing lived experience, insight, and heart into the room.

That's not "just" parenting—it's leadership.

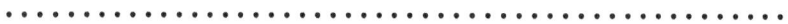

APPENDIX E

Recommended Resources

Support that reflects connection, regulation, and respect for neurodivergent lived experience.

Books That Align with CONNECT Values

◊ **The Whole-Brain Child – *Daniel J. Siegel & Tina Payne Bryson*** Neuroscience meets real-life parenting with clear strategies to support emotional regulation.

◊ **Unconditional Parenting – *Alfie Kohn*** Challenges behaviourist models and encourages respect, relationship, and autonomy.

◊ **The Book Between – *Sarah Ockwell-Smith*** Compassionate guidance for parenting tweens with emotional understanding and connection.

◊ **Nurturing Your Young Autistic Person – *Jude Morrow*** A neurodiversity-affirming book focused on acceptance, understanding, and practical strategies.

◊ **Super Powers for Parents – *Dr. Stephen Briers*** Helps parents co-regulate with their children by building emotional awareness and connection.

Deeper Reading & Research (for those who want more)

◊ **Polyvagal Theory - *Stephen Porges*** On how the nervous system shapes safety, regulation, and connection.

◊ **The Boy Who Was Raised as a Dog - *Bruce Perry & Maia Szalavitz*** Trauma-informed insights on safety, co-regulation, and healing.

◊ **The Body Keeps the Score - *Bessel van der Kolk*** How stress and trauma live in the body and the importance of regulation.

◊ **Sensory Integration and the Child - *A. Jean Ayres*** Foundational work on sensory processing.

◊ **The Out-of-Sync Child - Carol Stock Kranowitz** Accessible overview of sensory differences for families.

◊ **Raising a Sensory Smart Child - *Biel & Peske*** Everyday strategies for supporting sensory needs at home.

◊ **The Double Empathy Problem - *Damian Milton*** Research highlighting the two-way nature of communication differences.

Podcasts & Audio-Visual Tools

◊ **Neurodivergent Insights Podcast – *Dr. Megan Anna Neff*** Offers rich, identity-affirming insights into autism, ADHD, and lived neurodivergent experience.

◊ **AVUK Training – *Auditory Verbal UK*** Clear, accessible training for professionals and parents, available online and face-to-face.

◊ **Carol Gray's Social Stories** A framework for supporting understanding, especially when adapted with respectful, affirming language.

◊ **Neuro Embrace Community - *Madeline Woolgar*** A gentle, validating support space for parents of neurodivergent children, rooted in respect and co-regulation.

Websites & Organisations to Explore

◊ **AVUK (Auditory Verbal UK)** Evidence-based early intervention grounded in playful, meaningful connection. **www.avuk.org**

◊ **SENDIAS** Offers impartial, legally informed advice to parents navigating education systems in the UK. **www.councilfordisabledchildren.org.uk (> About > Our Networks >** Information, Advice and Support Services Network **>** Find your local IAS service)

◊ **Not Fine In School** Advocacy and understanding for children with emotionally based school avoidance. **www.notfineinschool.co.uk**

◊ **Contact** A national charity for families with disabled children, offering emotional and legal support. **www.contact.org.uk**

◊ **PDA Society** Offers information, lived experience insights, and community resources for those with a PDA profile. **www.pdasociety.org.uk**

◊ **Autistic Girls Network** Raises awareness and provides support for autistic girls, including around late diagnosis and masking. **www.autisticgirlsnetwork.org**

Want to share additional aligned resources which have really helped your family (or you have used in your practice)? I'd love to hear from you!

www.connectcommunicationtherapy.com

Evaluating Advice Through a Neurodiversity-Affirming Lens

Not every resource, professional approach, or programme will align with your values.

Here are a few things to look for:

- Does it respect autonomy and difference, rather than aiming to "fix" the child?

- Is the goal *connection and communication*, not compliance or correction?

- Does it include lived experience voices—especially autistic, ADHD, deaf and/or disabled perspectives?

- Are strategies based on co-regulation, relationship, and real-life—not rigid systems or rewards?

· ·

Note: If a resource leaves you feeling judged, overwhelmed, or disconnected from your child—it may not be the right fit.

Trust your instincts.

You are your child's safest person, and the right support will honour that.

· ·

APPENDIX F

Regulation Strategies for Real Life

Real tools. Real moments. Rooted in connection.

. . . .

Every child has their own sensory profile. Some seek more input, some avoid it, and some fluctuate between the two. This appendix shares regulation strategies that families have found helpful across ages and situations.

The aim isn't to "calm down" a child, but to create safety, stability, and shared connection. Regulation is about feeling safe, settled, and supported—together.

(These ideas are drawn from everyday practice with families, informed by principles of sensory integration. For tailored assessment or intervention, families are advised to consult an Occupational Therapist with advanced training in Sensory Integration. See also: Ayres; Biel & Peske; Kranowitz.)

By Sensory Need

Movement Seekers (vestibular/proprioceptive)

TRY THIS
- ► Jumping games (trampoline, sofa bounces, star jumps)
- ► Rolling up in a blanket or duvet burrito
- ► Animal walks (bear, crab, frog)
- ► Wheelbarrow races or carrying heavy bags

Sound Seekers / Sound Sensitive

TRY THIS
- ► Predictable music playlists (e.g. same "get ready" song each morning)
- ► Noise-cancelling headphones or ear defenders
- ► White noise or nature sounds
- ► Singing or humming together to match breath

By Sensory Need (cont.)

Touch Seekers / Touch Sensitive

[TRY THIS] ► Weighted lap pad or soft compression vest

► Lotion massage or brushing routines

► Fidget items with different textures

► Soft, tag-free clothing and favourite fabrics

Smell Seekers / Sensitive to Smell

[TRY THIS] ► Scented putty or scratch-and-sniff stickers

► Child-safe essential oil rollerballs (low scent)

► Avoid strong detergents or overpowering sprays

By Everyday Context

For Car Journeys

- ► Favourite snack or chew toy
- ► Visual countdown: *"3 songs, then we're there"*
- ► Small bag of sensory tools (pop toy, squishy, sunglasses)
- ► Rhythm games or tapping to music

For School Transitions

- ► Movement before school (e.g. *"Five jumps to the door"*)
- ► Predictable goodbye script or connection object (e.g. *"One squeeze, one kiss"*)
- ► Use Talking Ahead: *"First coat, then car, then school"*
- ► Drop-off buddy system or key adult handover

By Everyday Context

Before Bedtime

- Dim lights and soften sounds early
- Deep pressure cuddle, blanket burrito, or body sock
- Shared breathing: *"In through your nose, blow out the candles"*
- Audio story or calming playlist
- Visual countdowns (bath - PJs - story - sleep)

By Age & Communication Style

Toddlers & Pre-Speakers

- ► Simple action songs and nursery rhymes
- ► Blowing bubbles for slow breathing and eye tracking
- ► Lap games and bouncing on knees
- ► Visual supports for "all done", "more", "stop" and "go"

School-Age Children

- ► Offer regulation choices: *"Stretch or squish?"*
- ► Talk about body cues: *"Is your engine too fast, too slow, or just right?"*
- ► Rhythm games, silly walks, or sensory breaks between tasks
- ► Encourage drawing or quiet building for wind-down

By Age & Communication Style

Tweens & Teens

- ► Headphones, music, or movement breaks on their terms

- ► Practice advocacy scripts: *"I need a moment"*, *"I'm not ready yet"*

- ► Shared humour, games, or special interests as anchors

- ► Use self-awareness tools (energy check-ins, emotion scales)

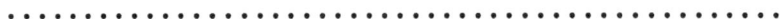

. . . .

Parent Tip:
Start with what you already know works for your child—don't try everything at once. Regulation is personal. One child may calm through movement, another through stillness. The goal isn't to eliminate dysregulation, but to provide safe exits and reliable ways back to connection.

Reflection Prompt

? What helps my child reset after a hard moment?

? Which daily routine tends to unravel— and which strategy above might help in that moment?

? What helps me regulate, so I can co-regulate with my child?

. . . .

Remember: Regulation is a shared process. It doesn't always look calm, but it should always feel safe.

If a strategy helps your child return to connection, it's working.

APPENDIX G

Supporting Non-Speaking Communicators

Connection doesn't wait for speech.

In the CONNECT Framework, communication is not a tick box. It's not something that starts with words—or ends with them. It begins with **connection, presence, and noticing.** For non-speaking children, this is especially true.

Whether a child uses gesture, movement, AAC, sound, or silence, they are already communicating. Our role is not to force speech—but to **listen differently**, to **model generously**, and to **respond warmly**.

What is "Non-Speaking"?

- A child might be non-speaking

  — temporarily (e.g. due to anxiety, trauma, or sensory shutdowns)

  — or consistently (e.g. due to motor planning challenges, apraxia, or developmental differences).

- Some people communicate **without words** for life—and that is a valid, whole form of communication.

What Communication Can Look Like Beyond Speech

Non-Speaking Behaviour	Possible Communication Function
Eye gaze or turning away	Interest / Avoidance
Reaching for an object or person	Request / Connection
Making a vocal sound or repeated noise	Protest / Attention / Sensory regulation
Smiling, frowning, or facial shifts	Emotion / Agreement / Discomfort
Hitting, biting, or bolting	Overwhelm / Escape / Need for regulation

Remember: All behaviour is communication. Our task is to interpret with kindness, not control.

CONNECT Strategies for Non-Speaking Communicators

Connection First

`TRY THIS` ► Sit beside them. Follow their lead. Don't demand eye contact or words.

► Use intonation, rhythm, and gesture to show you're listening.

Observe and Adapt

`?` ► What are they showing you with their body?

► Do they respond more with music? Movement? Visuals?

`TRY THIS` ► Adapt your language style: use pauses, repetition, and predictability.

CONNECT Strategies for Non-Speaking Communicators (cont.)

Natural Routines

TRY THIS
- ► Embed co-regulation and modelling in bath time, snack time, walking together.

- ► *"First socks, then shoes"*, even if they don't reply—language is still soaking in. Pause and give them time to process and engage.

Model Multi-Modal Communication

TRY THIS
- ► Use simple signs, objects, visuals, or AAC as you talk.

- ► Say then do or show, or point to pictures or icons while repeating: *"You want ball?"* [point to ball icon].

- ► Celebrate **all** communication—gestures, vocalisations, changes in breathing or body language.

Examples of Everyday Scripts (with or without AAC)

Situation	Honour and model words for *their* message
Reaching for snack	*"I want the **banana**"* [point to or offer picture of banana]
Pushing toy away	*"Let's say **'No thank you.'** That's okay."*
Rocking or flapping	*"We're **excited!** I see that!"*
No response	*"I'm still here. We don't need words right now."*
During AAC modelling	*"You say 'music' here."* [press or point to 'music']

For Extended Family, Professionals, and Friends

TRY THIS

→ *"He understands more than he can say."*

→ *"She's learning language in her own time."*

→ *"They use their body and eyes to communicate—watch closely."*

→ *"We respond to all communication, not just words."*

. . . .

Final Thought: Non-speaking does not mean non-communicative.

It means we must *slow down, tune in,* and *build communication together*— through rhythm, relationship, and shared joy.

Connection is the first language. Communication grows from there.

APPENDIX H

Scripts for Siblings, Grandparents & Extended Support

Helping others support your child in connection-first, relationship-rich ways.

....

Sometimes, the people who love our children most aren't sure how to help—or feel unsure when communication or behaviour doesn't follow expected patterns. This appendix is here to **equip you with gentle language** you can use to help others understand and support your child in ways that align with the CONNECT philosophy.

These are not scripts to memorise. They're conversation starters to help extended family, friends, siblings, and professionals come alongside you—without pressure, without judgement, and always with connection first.

Scripts for Grandparents & Extended Family

TRY THIS → *"He understands more than he can say right now—he just needs time and connection."*

→ *"You don't need to quiz or correct her. Just play alongside her and talk about what you're doing."*

→ *"He might not look at you or answer, but he's listening. You being there helps him feel safe."*

→ *"If she walks away, it's not rude—it's how she shows she needs space. She'll come back when she's ready."*

→ *"We're focusing on connection and regulation first—not speech or behaviour goals."*

· ·

Tip: Offer a few "safe" activities together, like...

- ► Stirring something in the kitchen
- ► Watering plants
- ► Looking at photos together
- ► Sitting quietly with music or sensory toys

· ·

Scripts for Siblings

TRY THIS → *"Your brother doesn't use many words, but he does tell us things in other ways. You're really good at noticing."*

→ *"She might flap or spin when she's excited. That's just how her body shows big feelings."*

→ *"You don't have to teach him. Just playing with him helps so much."*

→ *"When you sit with her and include her, even if she doesn't join in, she feels that."*

→ *"We're all learning together how to understand what your sibling needs. Thanks for being part of the team."*

· ·

Tip: Help siblings feel involved...

► Let them lead one game with a shared goal (e.g. build a tower together)

► Create a shared quiet space they can go to **with or without** their sibling

► Offer solo time with you, too—it matters

· ·

Scripts for Friends, Babysitters, and Occasional Visitors

TRY THIS → *"He might not answer questions, but you can still talk to him like you would anyone else."*

→ *"We try not to say things like 'good listening'—we focus more on connection."*

→ *"If she seems overwhelmed, you can just pause and give her space. No need to keep talking."*

→ *"It's okay if he doesn't play the 'usual' way. Let him take the lead—he'll show you so much."*

Scripts for Professionals Who Are New to Your Child

TRY THIS

→ *"We're using a connection-first framework called CONNECT—it's about relationship, regulation, and communication as an outcome."*

→ *"Please feel free to wait and watch before jumping in. My child often needs time to process information and feel safe."*

→ *"We're focusing on natural routines and real-life interaction—so what might look like 'doing nothing' is actually very purposeful."*

→ *"She communicates with her eyes and actions more than her voice. Watch her face—you'll see so much."*

→ *"I'm happy to share what works at home if that's helpful. It's not about getting it perfect—it's about noticing and responding."*

When You're Not Sure What to Say...

TRY THIS → *"We're doing things differently—and it's really helping."*

→ *"Thanks for being open to learning about what supports our child best."*

→ *"There's not one right way. But connection always comes first for us."*

→ *"If something feels hard, it's okay to ask or pause. We're all learning."*

. . . .

Final Thought: Your child's world expands when others are willing to meet them where they are. And often, they just need a little language—and a lot of permission—to do it differently.

Connection isn't a method. It's a mindset.

And the more people who share it, the safer our children feel.

APPENDIX I

Language for Reports, Forms & Advocacy Documents

Writing that reflects the whole child—not just their challenges.

. . . .

We often have to describe our children in reports, reviews, and funding applications. But many systems default to deficit-based language—words that don't reflect your child's strengths, personality, or what truly helps them thrive.

This appendix offers **gentle alternatives** that honour the CONNECT philosophy: human-first, neurodiversity-affirming, and focused on what supports regulation, connection, and communication.

Reframing Common Phrases

Traditional Language	CONNECT-Aligned Alternative
"Non-compliant with adult direction"	"Expresses autonomy through selective engagement"
"Refuses to follow instructions"	"Needs relational support to feel safe engaging with adult-led tasks"
"Limited verbal output"	"Communicates using multi-modal strategies including gesture, facial expression, and vocalisation"
"Demand avoidant"	"Highly sensitive to demands; benefits from autonomy, trust, and co-regulation"
"Delayed speech and language"	"Developing communication skills at their own pace, supported by real-life routines and shared experiences"

Traditional Language	CONNECT-Aligned Alternative
"Sensory issues"	"Distinct sensory profile; responds positively to sensory-aware environments"
"Displays challenging behaviour"	"Communicates distress through behaviour when dysregulated or overwhelmed"
"Unable to work independently"	"Thrives with co-regulation and relational scaffolding during learning tasks"
"Struggles with transitions"	"Benefits from clear, predictable routines and transition support strategies"

Positive, Strengths-Based Descriptions

EG **Instead of:**

"He avoids eye contact and doesn't engage with peers."

TRY THIS **Try:**

"He connects through side-by-side play and shared interests, and expresses preference for low-pressure social interaction."

....

EG **Instead of:**

"She is very anxious and becomes distressed in busy environments."

TRY THIS **Try:**

"She experiences sensory and emotional overload in busy spaces and thrives in calm, predictable environments with trusted adults."

Tips for Writing with Respect and Purpose

✓ **Lead with connection:** Start with what makes the child feel safe and seen.

✓ **Describe what helps:** Include co-regulation strategies, routines, or sensory tools that support success.

✓ **Avoid deficit-only labels:** Describe behaviours in the context of need—not as "problems".

✓ **Include the child's perspective where possible:** "He lets us know he's not ready by..."

✓ **Highlight natural learning:** Describe how growth happens in real-life routines, not just interventions.

Useful Phrases to Include in Forms or Reports

✍ "We are following the CONNECT Framework, which places connection, regulation, and everyday interaction at the heart of communication."

✍ "Progress for our child looks like increased safety, trust, and self-expression—in any form."

✍ "Our approach is relationship-based and neurodiversity-affirming; we seek support that reflects this."

✍ "Strategies that focus on shared routines, co-regulation, and responsive environments have been most effective."

✍ "We are not prioritising spoken output alone—we are supporting whole-child communication."

Final Thought: Words matter. The language we use shapes how others see our children—and how our children see themselves.

Let's write in a way that reflects who they truly are: whole, worthy, and deeply communicative in their own right.

Let your language advocate for the child, not just describe them.

APPENDIX J

Supporting Your Young Person into Employment & Purpose

From shared routines to meaningful roles—growing connection through contribution.

. . . .

As your child grows, you may begin to think about **what's next.** Whether that means supported employment, volunteering, self-employment, or simply discovering interests and strengths, the CONNECT Framework can continue to guide the process.

. . . .

This appendix isn't a checklist—it's a **relational pathway.** A way to think about how we prepare neurodivergent young people for meaningful roles in the world by prioritising **safety, confidence, joy, and belonging.**

Stage 1: Notice What Brings Joy and Energy

💡 **"What lights them up?"**

⊕ Start here. Before careers. Before skills. Before CVs. Focus on what they love, return to, or feel proud of.

✅ **Watch for signs of flow:**

- Long attention span during certain activities

- Repetition or deep interest (e.g. trains, maps, animals, tools)

- Joyful participation—without being prompted

☑ **Gather information gently:**

→ *"I've noticed you always help with the garden—what do you like about it?"*

→ *"You've been drawing logos lately... should we look at how real companies design theirs?"*

. . . .

Tip: Create a *Strengths & Interests Scrapbook*—with photos, drawings, or examples.

. . . .

Stage 2: Build Skills Inside Trusted Routines

🙂 **"Try it where they already feel safe."**

➡️ We don't need to simulate the real world with pressure and demands. We can embed contribution into real life.

EG **Examples:**

- ► Helping prep a favourite meal

- ► Creating shopping lists or packing bags for a trip

- ► Sorting or organising items (books, recycling, pet care)

💭 **Remember: This isn't about compliance—it's about confidence, competence, and feeling useful in a way that's valued.**

Stage 3: Bridge to Community— Gently and Supportively

♥ **"Go slow. Go together."**

For many neurodivergent young people, stepping into unfamiliar spaces is dysregulating. **Scaffold it** through shared visits, co-working, and predictable structure.

TRY THIS **Ideas:**

- Volunteering *with* a parent or mentor for a set time

- Starting with short visits to a future workplace

- Practising scripts or routines for interactions (e.g. *"I'm here to help restock"*, *"Where would you like me?"*)

📌 **Tip: Choose places that reflect your child's values and needs—quiet spaces, nature-based roles, hands-on tasks, low-verbal environments.**

Stage 4: Create a Safety Net for Success

✓ Success isn't doing something independently—it's **being supported in a way that honours how you work best.**

TRY THIS **Consider:**

- A named mentor or job coach
- Flexible hours or sensory-friendly schedules
- Pre-agreed communication supports (e.g. written instructions, visuals, quiet space access)

Help your young person practise self-advocacy language, like:

→ *"I need a short break when it gets loud."*

→ *"Can I write that down instead of saying it out loud?"*

→ *"It helps me when I have one task at a time."*

Stage 4: Create a Safety Net for Success (cont.)

Document supports in a 'This Is Me' Profile—not a diagnosis sheet, but a summary of:

- ✓ What helps me feel safe
- ✓ How I like to communicate
- ✓ What I'm good at and proud of

Supporting Language for Parents & Supporters

→ *"We're not rushing independence—we're growing interdependence."*

→ *"My young person has a lot to offer, with the right supports in place."*

→ *"Success for them looks like contribution, not just employment."*

→ *"We're focused on purpose, not pressure."*

. . . .

Final Thought: There is no one path. Some young people will find joy in freelance projects, some in part-time roles, some in volunteering at a farm, or building a tiny business from home.

What matters is that their gifts are recognised, their needs are respected, and their sense of self is preserved.

Work should never come at the cost of wellbeing. Contribution should always begin with connection.

. . . .

APPENDIX K

Everyday CONNECT in Action

Real stories, real moments.

....

The CONNECT Framework isn't about adding more to your to-do list. It's about noticing differently, responding differently, and finding connection in the ordinary. **Here are a few examples across ages and themes that show CONNECT in practice (all names changed to protect privacy).**

....

Toddler: Snack Time

💡 *Offering choice, reducing pressure*

🌱 Ella, aged two, often threw her cup across the room at snack time. Her parents felt stuck between giving in or bracing for another meltdown.

Together, we tried a simple adaptation. Instead of presenting the cup without words, her mum held up two options and said, *"First choose... then drink."* Ella pointed, smiled, and reached.

The cup stayed on the table. The meltdown never arrived. A tiny shift in language and predictability turned a daily battle into a moment of connection.

Toddler: The Shoes & the Coat

Pip had just discovered the magic of using her voice more often. She loved pointing, showing, and watching closely to figure out what adults meant. Most of her understanding came from seeing, not hearing.

One morning, her mum tried something different. Instead of pointing to the hallway or holding up Pip's coat, she simply said:

"Pip, go and get your shoes... and your coat."

No gesture. No clue. Just gentle, listening-only language.

Pip froze for a moment. You could almost see her thinking: *Wait... I didn't see anything. What does she mean?* Her eyes darted to Mum's face, checking for a hint.

Mum just smiled and waited.

And slowly — almost proudly — Pip toddled off. She didn't get it right first time. She came back with one shoe and a toy. Mum laughed kindly, repeated the instruction, and Pip tried again.

This time she came back with both shoes and the coat trailing behind her like a little cape.

Her arrival was pure triumph.

This wasn't about shoes or coats.

It was Pip learning to **listen,** not just watch.

To trust that words can guide her, even when the world gives no pictures.

Tiny moments like this turn the volume up on a toddler's auditory world — and they matter far more than we realise.

Toddler: The Tap-Tap Game

💡 *Serve-and-return, playful reciprocity*

🌱 Arlo had a favourite game in therapy — he'd tap the table with one finger, very softly, and then look up at me as if to say, *"Your turn."*

So I tapped back.

Tap.

Tap-tap.

Tap.

Arlo grinned, realising we'd started a rhythm together. Soon he added a sound — a tiny *"ba!"* — and waited.

So I echoed:

"Ba!"

His whole body lit up. Not because we were practising speech, but because he felt **heard, matched,** and **important.**

For toddlers like Arlo, games like this are the beginning of language.

Before the words, there is rhythm.

Before conversations, there is turn taking through imitation.

Before confidence, there is connection.

And every tap and "ba!" is a brick in that foundation.

Toddler: The Red Puzzle Piece Under the Table

Stretching auditory comprehension

During a home visit, Lena was playing with a puzzle. One piece — the red one — had disappeared under the table.

Her dad tried something new:

"Lena, go and get the red piece that's under the table."

This was a longer instruction than she was used to. Usually she was guided by gestures or familiar routines. But today, Dad wanted to stretch her listening gently.

Lena paused, squinted, and then dropped to her hands and knees, peering under the table.

Out came the red piece — dusty but victorious.

She beamed.

Dad beamed back.

And in that moment, Lena learnt that long strings of words can make sense — even when they're hidden under the table.

Toddler: The Fizzy Body

Big feelings with boundaries

Jonah was having one of those days where his body felt too big for him. His limbs were fast, his feelings even faster.

He wanted raisins. Then he didn't.

He wanted Mum. Then he pushed her away.

He wanted to throw the cushions just to release the fizz.

When he hit out in frustration, Mum knelt down, calm and steady:

*"I'm not going to let you hit me. But you **can** hit this cushion."*

She placed a big, soft cushion in front of him and stayed close.

Jonah thumped it hard — once, twice, three times — and then collapsed into her arms, the storm passing as suddenly as it began.

He wasn't being naughty.

He was overwhelmed.

And Mum showed him: *Your feelings are big, but you're safe. I'm here.*

Toddlers learn regulation through our nervous systems, not our explanations. Jonah didn't need a lecture; he needed a boundary wrapped in connection.

Toddler: I Have Another Idea!

Advocacy language

Theo was playing with cars with his grandma. She set up a ramp, but Theo pushed it aside and tried to build a bridge instead.

When Grandma tried to redirect him, he frowned and said: *"No... my turn."*

He meant: *I have a different plan.*

But he didn't yet have the language for that.

So Grandma gently modelled:

"That's one idea... but you've got another idea."

Theo's face changed.

He looked at his bridge with pride — *Yes. That's it. Another idea.*

For toddlers, these tiny scripts shape everything: confidence, flexibility, negotiation, self-advocacy. It wasn't about the cars or the ramp. It was about giving Theo the words to express himself clearly, kindly, and with courage.

Toddler: The Missing Word

💡 *Modelling grammar without correcting*

🌱 Beau held up a picture he'd drawn and declared proudly:

"I made a small!"

His mum almost corrected him — *"a small what?"* — but she stopped herself and instead modelled:

"You made a small one! Wow, look at that!"

Beau repeated, *"Small one!"* and giggled as though he'd cracked a secret code.

No pressure.

No "wrong" or "right".

Just gentle modelling that filled in the pieces without breaking his flow.

Toddlers grow grammar the same way they grow everything else — by absorbing what they hear in moments of real joy.

Toddler: Quiet for Baby

💡 *Preparing for transition*

🌱 Jasper was expecting a baby sibling soon. His parents were nervous — he was excitable, loud, and impulsively affectionate.

They practised with a doll first. Jasper rocked it wildly, kissed its face, then tried to feed it crisps.

Instead of correcting him, his dad whispered playfully:

"Shhh... gentle hands for baby."

Jasper froze, then softened his touch dramatically, stroking the doll's head with exaggerated care. He whispered,

"Baby sleep."

It became a game — loud hands, quiet hands; big voice, tiny voice. Jasper loved it.

By the time the real baby arrived, he already had a playful, embodied understanding of gentleness that no rulebook could teach.

School Age: Playground Conflict

Talking Ahead script

Daniel came back from break with fists clenched and tears in his eyes. *"They never let me play,"* he muttered.

The teacher almost reminded him of the rules—but we paused. What game was it? Football.

I crouched down and said, ***"That sounds tough. You wanted in, and it felt like you were shut out."***

He nodded.

We practised a Talking Ahead script for the next day: ***"First I'll ask if I can join. Then, if it's too hard, I'll find my buddy or ask the teacher to help."***

It wasn't about fixing football. It was about giving Daniel a sense of safety and choice.

School Age: The Hiding Game

Double empathy

During a session, Maya told me about a game she sometimes plays with two friends. She explained it very openly, without any sense that she was doing something wrong — just describing the way things often unfold.

She said that when all three of them are together, she and her closest friend sometimes suggest playing hide-and-seek. They encourage the third girl to go and hide first... and once she's hidden, Maya and her friend wander off and play together instead.

There was no malice in the way she told the story. No smirk, no sense of "we got away with something."

Just a child calmly explaining a social workaround she and her friend have developed — a way to make things feel

295

easier, quieter, or less overwhelming when the dynamic of three feels too much.

This is such an important moment in CONNECT work, because it highlights how **empathy works both ways.**

On the surface, yes, the third child is being excluded.

But underneath, Maya is communicating something just as real:

→ *"I get overwhelmed in a group of three."*

→ *"I find this friend's energy hard to manage."*

→ *"I don't know how to say I need space."*

Children rarely say these things directly.

Instead, the behaviour says it for them.

So rather than stepping in with correction or judgement, we slow down and get curious:

- ► What felt hard in that moment?

- ► What was she needing?

- ► What was her friend needing?

- ► And what might the third child have been feeling as she hid, waiting for the game to begin?

Empathy here isn't about blame.

It's about gently helping Maya widen the frame:

→ *"Yes, it sounds like it felt calmer with just the two of you."*

And also:

→ *"How do you think she felt, hiding and waiting?"*

→ *"What would help you ask for space in a kinder, clearer way?"*

→ *"What helps you when you feel overwhelmed?"*

This is where the real learning happens — not in punishment, but in supported reflection.

It's about helping Maya notice her own regulation needs and connect with someone else's experience at the same time.

It's also about giving her tools for boundaries that don't require avoidance or exclusion.

Because empathy isn't a one-way street.

It's something we grow by holding two truths at once: **your feelings matter, and so do theirs.**

Teen: Overloaded After School

Rhythm & predictability

Sophie, 14, often slammed her bag down and stormed upstairs the minute she got home. Her parents worried she was shutting them out.

Instead of confronting her, they started observing her rhythm. School drained her, and she needed recovery time before re-engaging. They adapted their expectations: no immediate questions, no chores right away.

They added a predictable phrase: ***"I'm here when you're ready."***

Within weeks Sophie began coming downstairs on her own terms to share about her day.

CONNECTION BEFORE CORRECTION ~ Aidan

Aiden walked into the room with his hands buried deep in his sleeves, shoulders tight, eyes scanning for exits more than people. The teacher mouthed, *"He won't manage anything today."*

But Aiden didn't need managing.
He needed somewhere safe to land.

So instead of a task, I sat beside him on the floor and began building a small tower of magnetic tiles. No questions. No prompting. Just slow, predictable movement.

After a minute, he nudged one tile into place.

Two minutes later, he quietly said, *"My brother broke my other one at home."*

Ten minutes later, we were problem-solving a sequencing task he had refused all week.

Connection didn't warm him up for the learning. Connection *was* the learning.

OBSERVE & ADAPT ~ Jasmine

Jasmine looked "off task" in science. She stared at her lap, pencil untouched, worksheet pristine. Hood up. A teaching assistant whispered, *"She's not with us this afternoon."*

But when I sat beside her, I noticed her eyes flicking back and forth in tiny micro-movements. She was silently rehearsing every answer — trying to perfect it before daring to write.

Her difficulty wasn't comprehension.
It was perfectionism.

So we adapted the demand:

Instead of *"Write four reasons"*, I said, *"Circle the one you want to **talk about** first."*

She circled immediately.

Once the pressure was off, she wrote three full sentences.

Observation isn't passive.
It's the gateway to adaptation.

NATURAL LANGUAGE OPPORTUNITIES ~ Leo

Leo shut down in class the moment the lesson activity was placed in front of him. No amount of questioning coaxed a response.

But when he helped set up the art trolley — pouring water, squeezing paint, wiping tables — the language flowed:

"Too much red!"

"It's spilling!"

"Wait, I need another cup!"

Not prompted. Not pulled.

Just happening.

Some children don't need more questions. They need meaningful moments.

NEURODIVERSITY-AFFIRMING PRACTICE ~ Imogen

Imogen dreaded lunchtime. The hall was too loud, too bright, too unpredictable. Adults kept encouraging her to *"be brave"* or *"push through"*, but her body simply couldn't.

When I asked what it felt like, she said:

"It's like someone turns all the sounds up but none of them make sense."

So we made some small adjustments:

- ► five minutes of quiet corridor transition
- ► noise-dampening headphones
- ► visual schedule for the lunch queue
- ► permission to sit at the end of the table

Within weeks, she began chatting more, eating more, and even joining playground games.

Support didn't change *Imogen*.

Support changed the environment so she could be herself.

PRE-STRUCTURING LANGUAGE TO REDUCE OVERWHELM ~ Kieron

Kieron was brilliant at ideas but froze whenever he was asked open questions like *"Tell me what happened in the story."*

His breathing quickened, his eyes darted, and he'd mutter, *"I don't know"*, even though he did.

So we pre-structured the whole task with a simple verbal scaffold — always the same:

"First...
Then...
After that..."

I modelled the pattern first, keeping my voice slow and rhythmic.

He copied the pattern, then added his own details.

Within a few weeks, he could retell whole sequences, not because his memory suddenly improved, but because the structure supported his working memory, anxiety, and processing.

The right scaffold doesn't replace the child's thinking.

It frees it.

EMOTIONAL REGULATION AS A FOUNDATION FOR COMMUNICATION ~ Jax

Jax was having "off days" more often — tight shoulders, clipped answers, a readiness to misread tone or assume he was in trouble. Staff thought it was attitude; I knew it was overload.

During a transition between lessons, he muttered, *"Everyone's in my way."*

That was the moment.

Instead of pushing on, I named what I saw gently:

"Your body looks busy."

He exhaled — the long, shaky kind.

We took 60 seconds to reset using his chosen strategy:

Feet planted, slow breath in, longer breath out.

Only after his body settled did he attempt the reading task.

And he managed it brilliantly.

Language didn't fail him.

His nervous system needed support first.

EXECUTIVE FUNCTION & NARRATIVE ORGANISATION ~ Callum

Callum's stories were a whirlwind — brilliant ideas but no sequence, no markers, and no way to hold them together. Adults often said, "He goes off on tangents", when actually his brain was working faster than he could express.

So we used a "three-bead" chain — a physical object with three beads he slid along as he talked:

- ► Bead 1 — "Who are the characters?"

- ► Bead 2 — "What's the problem?"

- ► Bead 3 — "What's the solution?"

With something concrete to anchor him, a clearly scaffolded sequence, his narratives became clear, proud, and purposeful.

Sometimes executive function needs a handrail, not a correction.

EMPOWERED ADULT = EMPOWERED CHILD ~ Simran

Simran often melted down at the start of maths because she couldn't track multi-step instructions. Her teacher began using "auditory closure" phrasing instead of direct questioning:

"First we're going to look at the number line, then we're going to..."

"... add the jumps."

Simran filled in the final step confidently.

The teaching assistant later said, *"I thought she wasn't listening. Now I realise she just needed it worded differently."*

When adults feel empowered, children thrive.

Everyday CONNECT in Action: Reflection Prompt

? Which of these moments feels closest to your family's experience?

— A toddler who craves predictability?

— A school-age child struggling with peers or learning?

— A teen who seems distant?

? How could you try a small shift— observing differently, adapting gently, and putting connection first—in your own routines?

Glossary of Terms & Acronyms

Alternative and Augmentative Communication (AAC)

AAC includes tools such as signs, picture boards, symbols, and communication devices that support a child to make requests and share their messages and ideas when speech isn't there yet. They can often be used as a bridging strategy that leads to spoken words in the future. Within the CONNECT Framework, AAC is understood as a partnership tool — a way of reducing frustration, increasing connection, and giving children a reliable voice as their spoken language grows.

Auditory Verbal Therapy (AVT)

An evidence-based approach to developing spoken language in deaf children with hearing technology. AVT places parents at the centre, coaching them to embed listening and communication strategies into everyday routines.

Autonomy-Supportive Practice
A way of working that respects a child's need for choice, agency, and control. Instead of enforcing compliance, adults create safe, shared environments where children willingly engage.

Certified Member of the Royal College of Speech and Language Therapists (CertMRCSLT)
Professional registration status for UK speech and language therapists, confirming qualification and adherence to professional standards.

Co-Regulation
The process by which a caregiver helps a child regulate their emotions, body, and nervous system through presence, attunement, and supportive strategies. A foundation for communication and learning.

Communication as an Outcome of Regulation (CONNECT principle)
The idea that true communication happens when a child feels calm, safe, and regulated. Rather than pushing language, adults first focus on helping the child's nervous system settle.

Connection First (CONNECT principle)
The foundation of the CONNECT Framework.
Relationships and emotional safety come before
tasks, strategies, or language goals. Progress is
rooted in trust and presence.

CONNECT Framework®
A relational model developed by Susannah
Burden. CONNECT stands for:

- ▶ **C** – Connection First
- ▶ **O** – Observe and Adapt
- ▶ **N** – Natural Routines
- ▶ **N** – Neurodiversity-Affirming Practice
- ▶ **E** – Empowered Caregivers
- ▶ **C** – Communication as an Outcome of
  Regulation
- ▶ **T** – Togetherness

Deficit Lens
A way of viewing children that highlights what
they "lack" or "cannot do". The CONNECT
approach reframes this by focusing on strengths,
regulation, and context instead.

Dysregulation

When a child's nervous system is overwhelmed, leading to difficulty staying calm, focused, or engaged. Can show as meltdowns, shutdowns, or withdrawal. Regulation strategies restore safety.

Education, Health and Care Plan (EHCP)

A legal document in England outlining the support a child with special educational needs must receive across education, health, and social care.

Echolalia

The repetition of words or phrases, sometimes from TV, peers, or adults. Within CONNECT it's seen as a valid way of processing and communicating, not something to be extinguished.

Empowered Caregivers (CONNECT principle)

When parents and carers recognise their expertise, instincts, and role in their child's growth. Professionals act as partners and coaches, not gatekeepers.

Everyday Routines / Natural Routines (CONNECT principle)

Ordinary family activities (e.g. mealtimes, car journeys, bedtimes) used as rich opportunities for connection, language, and regulation.

Individual Education Plan (IEP)

A written plan that sets out the support and targets for a child with special educational needs, often used in schools.

Individual Support Plan (ISP)

A document outlining the additional help provided for a child, sometimes used as an alternative to or stepping stone towards an EHCP.

Listening and Spoken Language Specialist (LSLS)

An international certification for professionals specialising in developing listening and spoken language in children with hearing loss, trained through Auditory Verbal Therapy.

Neurodiversity

The natural variation in human brains and minds, including autism, ADHD, dyslexia, and more. It emphasises difference rather than deficit.

Neurodiversity-Affirming Practice (CONNECT principle)

An approach that honours difference without trying to "fix" the child. It adapts environments and expectations to meet the child's needs, rather than forcing conformity.

Observe and Adapt (CONNECT principle)

The practice of noticing a child's cues, rhythms, and signals, then flexibly adjusting responses to meet their needs in the moment.

Regulation

A state of balance where the nervous system is calm enough for connection and learning. Includes sensory, emotional, and physiological stability.

Sensory Profile

An individual's pattern of sensory needs (e.g. seeking movement, avoiding noise, preferring deep pressure). Understanding profiles helps adults create supportive environments.

Speech and Language Therapy / Therapist (SALT)

A professional service and role supporting communication, speech, language, and swallowing needs.

Strengths-Based Language

Describing children in terms of their abilities, preferences, and ways of connecting—rather than deficits or pathologies. Example: saying "communicates with sign language, or through gesture and expression" instead of "non-verbal".

Talking Ahead

A CONNECT strategy that uses simple "First... then..." scripts to prepare children for transitions and reduce anxiety by making events predictable.

Togetherness (CONNECT principle)

The recognition that children, families, and professionals thrive in community, not isolation. Growth happens in webs of support, not lone effort.

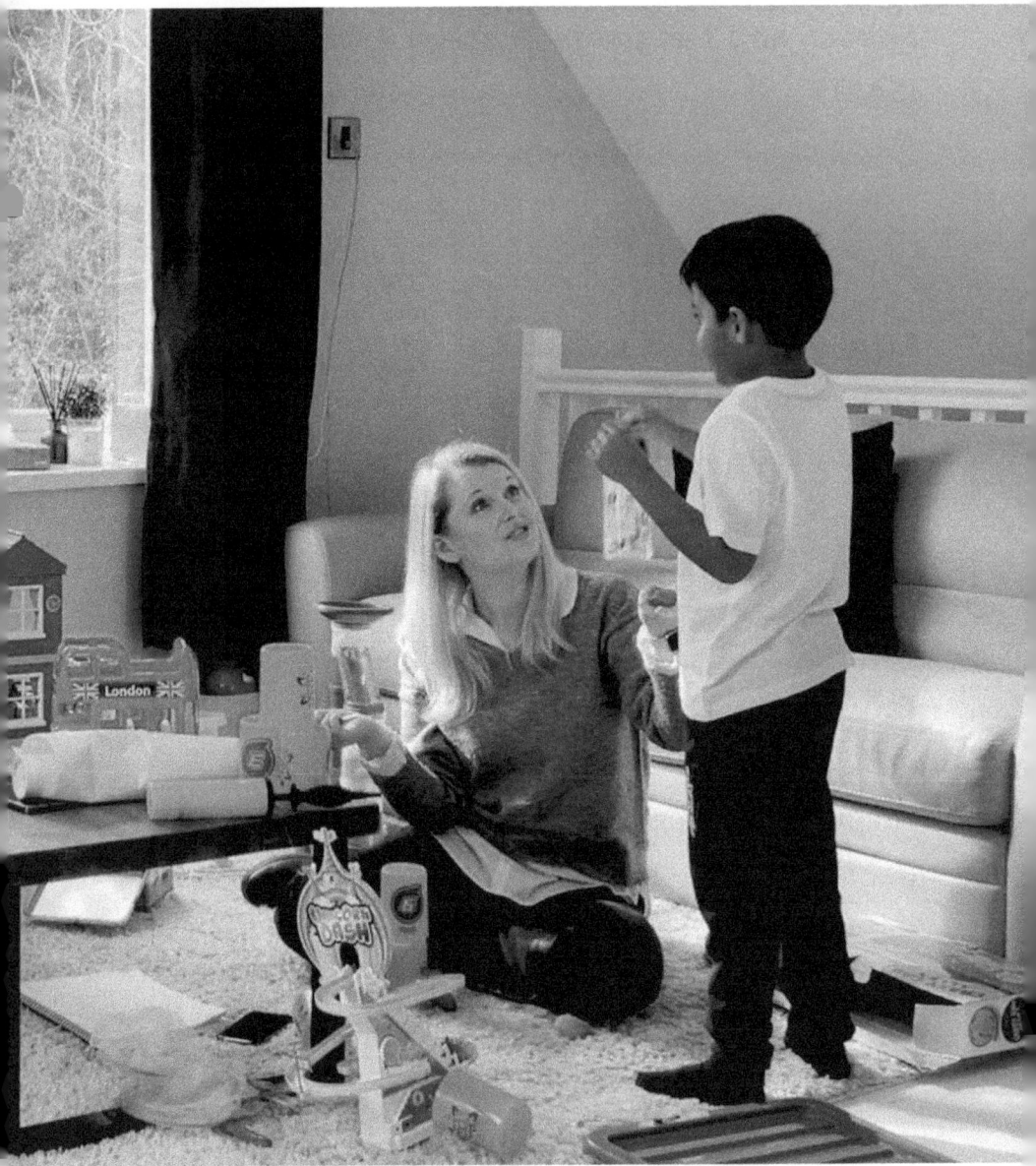

About the Author

Susannah Burden, BSc (Hons), CertMRCSLT, PgDip AVT, LSLS Cert AVT, is an independent Speech and Language Therapist and Certified Auditory Verbal Therapist with over 17 years' experience working alongside families, schools, and young people.

She founded Connect Communication Therapy Ltd to share her belief that true communication support begins not with drills or correction, but with connection, regulation, and trust.

As both a professional and a parent, Susannah understands the challenges families face. Her motivation for writing **CONNECT First** grew from years of listening to parents' stories, witnessing the power of everyday routines, and experiencing firsthand the difference that small shifts in perspective and practice can make.

She has presented both nationally and internationally on parent partnership and functional intervention, sharing practical, connection-first strategies that make a lasting difference.

Warm, practical, and rooted in real-life examples, her work continues to inspire both families and professionals to see communication not as a skill to be trained, but as a relationship to be nurtured.

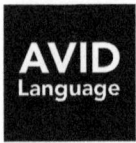

More books from AVID Language

AVID Languages publishes books for families with (and without) hearing loss.

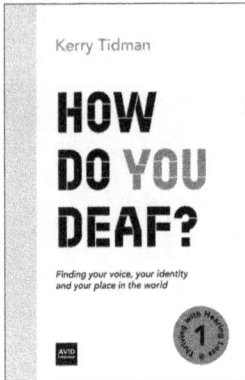

Kerry Tidman

HOW DO YOU DEAF?

Finding your voice, your identity and your place in the world

VOICES of HOPE

Inspirational stories of deaf children listening and speaking, told by their families

Supporting young people to find their identity, their voice (in whichever way they choose), and their place in the world.

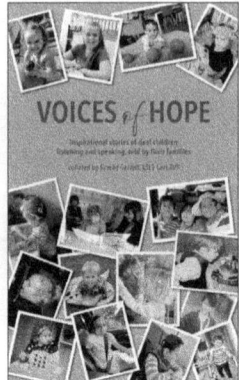

Personal accounts written by parents who have taught their profoundly deaf children to listen & speak.

View our full range of titles at www.avidlanguage.com/books

CONNECT FIRST
Published by AVID Language Limited, 3 Cam Drive, Ely, CB6 2WH, UK
First published in 2025

ISBN:
Paperback: 978-1-913968-98-4
Hardcover: 978-1-913968-99-1

Text © Susannah Burden 2025
Photo page 10 © Tanya & Ian Saunders 2019
Photo page 318 © Susannah Burden 2025
Editing, design & layout by Tanya Saunders for AVID Language

· ·

The CONNECT Framework®, developed by Susannah Burden, is a registered trademark of Connect Communication Therapy Limited.